SHAPING POLICY FOR LONG-TERM CARE

Learning from the Effectiveness of Hospital Swing Beds

SHAPING POLICY FOR LONG-TERM CARE

Learning from the Effectiveness of Hospital Swing Beds

Peter W. Shaughnessy

Health Administration Press
Ann Arbor, Michigan 1991

95 94 93 92 91   5 4 3 2 1

Library of Congress Cataloging-in-Publication Data

Shaughnessy, Peter.
    Shaping policy for long-term care : learning from the effectiveness of
hospital swing beds / Peter W. Shaughnessy.
        p.   cm.
    Includes bibliographical references.
    Includes index.
    ISBN 0-910701-71-7
    1. Long-term care of the sick—United States—Cost effectiveness.
2. Hospital swing beds—United States.   3. Medical policy—United
States.   I. Title.
    [DNLM: 1. Bed Conversion.   2. Health Facility Planning—United
States.   3. Health Policy—United States.   4. Long Term Care.   WX 162
S533s]
RA997.S48   1991   362.1'6'0973—dc20
DNLM/DLC for Library of Congress   91-7008 CIP

Health Administration Press
A division of the Foundation of the
    American College of Healthcare Executives
1021 East Huron Street
Ann Arbor, Michigan 48104-9990
(313) 764-1380

To Mother and Dad
for caring
and for your commitment to learning

Contents

Foreword

This superb book tells a success story. Over a period of roughly 20 years, swing-bed services in rural hospitals were developed, tested, refined, and adopted by more than 1,000 institutions. Swing-bed programs are now providing patients with demonstrably higher-quality care than they were likely to receive elsewhere, minimizing burdens on family members, and helping to ensure the survival of rural health care institutions, while still saving Medicare and Medicaid money. In an age when people have grown increasingly cynical about the capacity of anything, and certainly of any government program, to improve the lives of dependent populations, the success of swing beds is an important reminder that the system is capable of producing wins as well as losses.

The development of swing beds is also a success story in another sense. As Shaughnessy recounts so well, swing beds evolved in a process that proceeded, in a relatively orderly fashion, from an initial idea through preliminary experimentation, to more systematic testing, and then through successive iterations of modest expansion accompanied by thorough evaluation—a process that, in at least one sense, is still not complete and of which, in that regard, this book itself is a part. In other words, at least this once, the policymaking process behaved in what would appear to be a relatively rational way. An innovative idea was tested on a small scale; the apparent success of that innovation was followed by somewhat larger tests of the idea with minor variants, and those tests were closely monitored; new policy, based largely on the results of those tests, was adopted, but it too was implemented with some care and closely monitored. Such a process smacks more closely of introductory texts in policy analysis than of what most of us tend to think of as the real world, but at least in this case, it seems actually to have occurred, and to have worked rather well.

This "rational" process of policy evolution was made possible to a large extent by the high quality and total credibility of the evaluation research conducted at every stage by Shaughnessy and his colleagues. The author's modesty in this instance may be both becoming and understandable, but it affects his conclusions, at least a little, since the esteem in which he and his colleagues were held undoubtedly had a lot to do with the willingness of policymakers to take the conclusions of the research so seriously, and to support continuing research and evaluation efforts. By succinctly describing much of that research itself, Shaughnessy provides the reader with a chance to see first-hand what good policy research, of the type capable of influencing policy, should look like.

Shaughnessy is probably more sanguine than I about the likelihood that so rational a process can be frequently replicated—although, as he notes, his case speaks for itself. And there are other, at least partial, examples, perhaps the most prominent of which is the development of DRG-based hospital payment methods as part of a well-conceived program of reimbursement experiments. Perhaps more important, though, is the notion Shaughnessy advances so well, that ways can and must be found to ensure that, when good information is available, it gets injected into the policy process at a time and a place where it can do some good. Again, the strength of Shaughnessy's argument may be partially undercut by the ironical fact that his own research was of such atypically high quality, but the general proposition remains an important one, and one well worth pursuing.

Still, as much a success—in so many ways—as swing beds are, they are only the first step toward more systematic reform of long-term care services. Such reform is essential if we are to meet the needs of a burgeoning elderly population, especially of those on whom this book is focused, patients in need of what Shaughnessy, seeking to hack his way through the terminological thicket, has termed near-acute care. Two linchpins of such reform, as Shaughnessy well identifies them, are the adequate distinction between near-acute and chronic long-term care patients and services, and the clarification and expansion of Medicare's long-term care role; this second task may be made much easier to the extent that we are successful with the first. This book makes a number of specific suggestions about ways in which to proceed with the reform process, and one can only hope that policymakers are as responsive to them as they were to Shaughnessy's earlier recommendations about the development of the swing-bed program.

In a final irony, I can't resist noting that the success of swing beds was possible, in the first instance, in large part because of the failure of an earlier policy: the definition of an extended care facility benefit in the original Medicare legislation. To summarize a long story I have told elsewhere, what Shaughnessy now terms "near-acute" care was in fact covered as "extended care" when Medicare was first enacted. However, for a variety of reasons, the benefit was never effectively implemented. No one knew quite what "extended care" meant; facility models were few and hard to identify; the distinction between near-acute and chronic long-term care now so pivotal to effective policy development had not yet been made. More centrally, the world has changed in some very important ways since 1965: society has changed; medical technology has changed; most importantly, the tide of demographic change has now produced a demand for a level of service for which there probably just weren't enough potential patients in 1965. It's sometimes tempting to adopt the cynical view that there's really nothing new under the sun, that every ostensibly new idea in public policy was in fact first thought of by Thomas Jefferson or Ben Franklin or (in the medical world) Florence Nightingale, but in fact things change, and an idea that may make no sense in one generation is just the answer for another. Swing beds may well be an example.

This exemplary book thus contains multiple messages. It teaches a lot about how long-term care can be effectively delivered, and about how public policy should be changed to make more effective care more widely available to Medicare beneficiaries. It tells a lot about how to take a complex policy innovation and disseminate it to more than a thousand hospitals, many of them initially skeptical if not directly opposed. It has an awful lot to say about the uses of good research to make good policy. Most importantly, the very fact that it contains those and other messages demonstrates that policy, politics, analysis, and research can all come together for the benefit of people in need and us other citizens and taxpayers, at least once in a while.

Bruce C. Vladeck
President
The United Hospital Fund of New York

Preface

This is a story about two distinct, but interrelated, health policy issues. The first, and most important, entails the rather serendipitous discovery of a way to provide unusually effective health care to "near-acute care" patients, used in this book to mean long-term care patients with relatively intense medical and skilled nursing needs. Many such patients, if provided adequate health care, should be discharged home from a long-term care setting within several weeks of admission. Second, this is a story about the evolution of hospital swing beds—hospital beds that are used to provide both general hospital care and long-term care. The manner in which the swing-bed approach unfolded in the United States sheds considerable light on the essential ingredients of high-quality near-acute care.

Therefore, this book is concerned with how we might improve the way we provide near-acute care in the United States. This message is primarily conveyed by relating the history and effectiveness of swing-bed care. I hope the book documents only the first stage of our evolution in caring for near-acute care patients. My intent is to show that we can do considerably better than we are currently doing.

The novelty of the swing-bed story derives from the refreshingly rational manner in which the swing-bed idea grew to become a significant ingredient of our health care system in rural communities in the United States. At the same time, it clearly demonstrates the potential to improve the manner in which near-acute care is provided in our country. Nonetheless, enhancing near-acute care does not and should not depend exclusively on expanding swing-bed care as a primary vehicle for change, although further consideration of hospital swing beds in settings where they currently do not exist should probably be part of an agenda for such change.

The health policy lesson of the swing-bed program is simple but powerful: It is possible and effective to develop and improve health policy by implementing a new health care approach on a selected basis, evaluating its effects, determining its utility, suggesting needed refinements, and ultimately implementing a new national health care policy if the results of the experiment so dictate. My goal is for this message to unfold fairly naturally in these pages. In addition, the swing-bed movement in our country frames an unusually upbeat story that has a warm success to it that I have rarely encountered in professional life. In the second chapter, I have taken the liberty of occasionally intermixing the history of the program with a few incidents and illustrative cases intended to demonstrate the manner in which the swing-bed movement influenced, and was influenced by, particular individuals.

This book is intended for a relatively wide audience. It should be readable and interesting for health care providers, including hospital administrators and staff, nursing home administrators and staff, and physicians and nurses interested in the evolution of an approach to flexibly providing long-term care. For such readers, the contextual background of nursing home care and some aspects of hospital care are provided in the first chapter. This background is followed by an account of a fascinating growth process that began with a few hospitals in rural Utah. It also highlights the importance of two different philosophical approaches to long-term care: rehabilitative care and chronic or maintenance care. Each approach is critically important in the long-term care field, but we must be far more diligent than we have been in recognizing their differences and how to structure health policy in view of such differences.

Equally important, this book is written for health policymakers and students of health policy and health administration. The manner in which we semilogically tumbled to present-day policy in this area has some important lessons and perhaps will stimulate some serious and useful discussion on how the process of developing health policy might be rendered more rational. I would hope that people in my own field of health services research might find this book informative. Maybe it will contribute to the growing body of work on how to constructively influence the synergism between health policy and health services research. It is also my hope that the methods used in this research, especially those involved in measuring and analyzing the quality of care, will add to our ability to conduct health policy research.

Some lay readers might find the story interestingly optimistic. It begins with a reasonable idea targeted at helping the residents of rural communities. The idea and resultant program wend their way forward over approximately two decades, thanks to the involvement of a number of competent and reasonably objective people, to the point where the approach is now firmly in place and cost-effectively benefiting thousands of people daily.

In order to address a relatively wide audience, it was necessary to blend historical, anecdotal, policy, technical, and research facts and issues. Recognizing that certain types of details and information may be essential for some types of readers and unessential for others, a summary is presented at the end of each chapter. For example, the first summary might prove useful to some readers in skimming parts of Chapter 1 that deal with the historical and legislative background. In Chapters 5 and 6 on quality and cost, which present evidence justifying the cost effectiveness of near-acute care provided in swing beds, the summaries should also be helpful since these two chapters are necessarily research-oriented in nature. The summaries serve the important purpose of synthesizing the main points with a view toward supporting and highlighting the conclusions of the chapter.

The Chapter 5, 6, and 7 summaries are longer than others owing to the breadth of material covered. In view of the purposes of the chapter summaries—to make the book readable for a wide audience and to provide a contextual understanding of major points if one chooses to read selectively—some degree of redundancy is unavoidable between chapter text and summaries. However, this was judged to be offset by the advantages of providing summaries for purposes of review and reading efficiency—depending on the reader's preferences.

The text is divided into three parts. The first part (Chapter 1) provides the historical and policy backdrop for the rest of the book. Thereafter, Part II, which consists of Chapters 2–6, addresses the growth, evolution, and raison d'être of swing-bed care. Chapters 7 and 8 constitute Part III, which provides a discussion of several additional policy and health care issues in the long-term care field, with a view toward what we have learned and where we might go from here.

Acknowledgments

A large number of individuals have contributed either directly or indirectly to this book. I am most heavily indebted to Dr. Robert Schlenker. As friend and colleague, as well as coprincipal investigator and associate director of the Center for Health Services Research at the University of Colorado, Bob has been involved in nearly all phases of our research on hospital swing beds. Chapter 6 contains as much of his work as mine.

I appreciate the contributions of many colleagues at our research center with whom I have worked in researching the swing-bed movement over the past decade and a half. The conceptual and analytical contributions of Drs. David Hittle and Andrew Kramer were many and varied. Other research center staff who contributed include Shelda Harden, Inez Yslas, Marilyn Spencer, Patricia DeVore, Eileen Tynan, David Landes, Charles Huggs, Ann Jones, Walter Grant, Susan Foley, Richard Caston, Donna Vahling, Jon Stiles, Don Beck, Daniel Holub, Linda Breed, Kristin Paulson, Elizabeth Lutz, Arlene Woodson, Claudia Braunstein, Bettina Kurowski, Ann Trickler, Nancy Shanks, Jean Bell, Carol Pace, Christine Easton, Shinika Sykes, Daniel Jackson, Lynn Mason, Joseph McGloin, Jeffrey Amirani, Mary Pettigrew, Arthur McFarlane, Stephen Graff, and William Van Epps.

Several project officers and staff at the agencies that funded demonstrations and research work on the swing-bed program were actively involved in the program or its evaluation. These individuals include Herbert Silverman, Thomas Kickham, Spike Duzor, James Lubitz, James Baker, and Sandra Mikolaitis at the Health Care Financing Administration (HCFA) of the Department of Health and Human Services.

Program officers and staff from the Robert Wood Johnson Foundation (RWJF) who were involved in demonstration and evaluation efforts include Alan Cohen, Andrea Kabcenell, Jeffrey Merrill, Linda Aiken, Douglas Morgan, Peter Goodwin, Andrew Greene, Thomas Gregg, and

Lynne Long. I would especially like to acknowledge the suggestions and input of Alan Cohen, Herb Silverman, Andrea Kabcenell (the program officer for the grant that partially funded this book), and Tom Kickham in our research, and acknowledge their interest in the swing-bed program in general.

Two friends with whom I worked closely and who contributed significantly to the swing-bed story are Tony Kovner and Hila Richardson, who administered the RWJF's Rural Hospital Program of Extended Care Services out of New York City. A number of others involved in this program were also significant contributors to the material presented in this book: James Schuman, Donald Wilson, Jane Ford, Sarah Grim, Clark Crumm, Helen Smits, Gordon Russell, Mike Madden, Rheba de Tornay, Eldon Schumacher, and Francis Rogers.

I am extremely grateful to several professional colleagues who took the time to review and comment on the book in manuscript form. These include Marni Hall, Andrea Kabcenell, Andrew Kramer, Hila Richardson, Robert Schlenker, Herbert Silverman, and Bruce Vladeck. The revisions resulting from their comments not only rendered the text more readable, but they also increased the breadth and factual basis of the conclusions.

Several other friends and associates from the research, provider, and policy communities made important contributions to the evolution of hospital swing-bed care and near-acute care as discussed in this book. These include Jane Gibson, John Supplitt, Joshua Weiner, Lee Campbell, Dick Hager, Bruce Walter, Donald West, Neil Miller, Erwin Schumacher, William Scanlon, and Howard Freeman.

I am indebted to Robert Berg and Karen Fisher of the Center for Health Services Research for their editorial and substantive suggestions on the manuscript. Rob was especially helpful in the literature and background work necessary to place the swing-bed research in context. Cheryl Winston helped considerably in terms of technical and proofing work. Patricia DeVore played a significant technical and proofing role on much of our research work in the swing-bed field, and was also helpful in this area in the present book, as well as in preparation of maps and other figures. I appreciate the high-quality word processing done by Kay Jacobs, who entered and reentered the material for this book a number of times. Her contributions substantially enhanced the final manuscript.

In addition to carrying out their regular patient care duties, administrative and nursing personnel at swing-bed hospitals and nursing homes that received site visits as part of our many case studies and data collection programs willingly provided information and spent considerable time with research center staff members. Valuable assistance was provided by RWJF grantee hospitals and hospital associations; administrators, physicians, and nurses affiliated with swing-bed hospitals, comparison hospitals, nursing homes, and home health agencies; the Section for Small or Rural Hospitals of the American Hospital Association; state nursing home associations; personnel at HCFA central and regional offices; and staff members of various federal and state agencies involved in administering the swing-bed program, including Medicare Part A intermediaries, Medicare Part B carriers, peer review organizations, Medicaid fiscal agencies, state Medicaid offices, state licensure and certification agencies, and state planning agencies.

I am grateful for the organizational, administrative, and financial support provided by the Office of the Chancellor for Health Affairs at the University of Colorado Health Sciences Center. Without the assistance and endorsement of Chancellors Bernard Nelson and John Cowee, the research program whose results are documented here would not have been possible.

The staff at Health Administration Press were extremely helpful in improving the manuscript and expediting the publication of the book.

I am most appreciative of the support provided by the Robert Wood Johnson Foundation that enabled me to write this book. Equally important, I am grateful to both the Health Care Financing Administration and the Robert Wood Johnson Foundation for the funding provided to continue our research on hospital swing beds for the past 15 years. The conclusions reached and any recommendations made in this book are mine alone and do not necessarily reflect the official positions of these agencies. But it is a pretty safe bet that many of them really do. Otherwise the swing-bed program, and the insights it has given us on how to provide near-acute care, would not be part of our health care system today.

PART I

Introduction

CHAPTER 1

Policy Context

THE PEOPLE ISSUES

Rehabilitation Care versus Chronic Care

Overlooked in our society is the critical nature of hospital discharge as a key entry point into our long-term care delivery system for many people in the United States. For elderly patients especially, the recovery period after a hip fracture, stroke, or heart attack not only entails hospitalization, but it also frequently involves a nursing home stay. Depending on the condition of the patient, his or her recuperative power, and the extent to which the care received fosters independence versus dependence, the patient may never leave the nursing home. While it is at times appropriate for people to remain permanently in nursing homes, far too frequently the elderly in our country are either improperly assessed or improperly treated in view of their health care needs at the end of their hospital stay. Far too often such people never leave our nursing homes. At, or shortly after, hospital discharge, it is therefore of paramount importance for us to properly determine the precise types of long-term care needed to enhance independence and maximize the quality of an elderly person's life.

Out of sincere, but misdirected, sympathy and concern, elderly patients are often considered too frail to undergo a sustained period of rehabilitation directed toward achieving a lifestyle of greater independence and personal freedom. In some instances it is not misdirected concern, but neglect or inattentiveness to patient needs that brings this about. Some nursing home patients are overprovided services that render them more dependent than they should be over time (Gillick 1989). Assistance in functional areas such as bathing, dressing, and toileting are sometimes provided almost uniformly to certain types of nursing home residents, many of whom should be actively encouraged to become independent in these areas. This brings about what some have referred to as "learned helplessness" (Avorn and Langer 1982; Achenbaum 1978). The services many residents require should be characterized by an independence-fostering philosophy rather than a dependence-fostering philosophy.

Without doubt, we have many nursing home residents who permanently require basic services in order to function daily (the terms *residents* and *patients* are used interchangeably). As a society, we have an obligation to care for both the young and the old who require such services. However, we should also recognize that we have made many patients permanently dependent who should never have been so. It is not surprising that we have done this. The vast majority of care in nursing homes is provided by nurses aides who have limited, if any, training and experience in providing health care or long-term care prior to their first job with a nursing home. Such individuals are often employed at a minimum wage and taught how to bathe, dress, toilet, and feed a patient. It is often easier to bathe or feed patients, or even assist patients in getting to and from the commode, than it is to encourage patients to bathe or feed themselves, or get to and from the bathroom as independently as possible. Such encouragement often requires more time with the patient as well as persuasive and motivational skills. Patient failures at attempts to eat independently not only require additional work, but such work may be unpleasant for the aide.

Just how many patients have we made more dependent in this country than we should? No one really knows the precise number, but it is clear that this has happened and is continuing to happen. Certain types of providers of nursing home care, however, through greater emphasis on rehabilitation and restoration, have been able to substantially increase rates of discharge to independent living.

Nursing homes originated in this country to meet a bona fide need to care for patients, predominantly elderly, whose chronic care needs were such that they needed daily assistance in an institutional setting to survive. During the last 40 to 50 years, nursing homes have been given significant incentives by government to become involved in the provision of health care, rehabilitation care, and certain types of skilled nursing care. Nonetheless, the distinction between chronic (maintenance) care and rehabilitation care is immense. Not only do they require different qualifications and services, but they require a totally different orientation. A philosophy of rehabilitation care and a philosophy of maintenance care for chronically ill patients are as different as night and day.

Patients can be well-rehabilitated when they are properly assessed and provided the correct restorative and therapeutic services in an institutional setting (as well as in a noninstitutional outpatient or in-home setting in some instances)—and this is good. Analogously, properly assessing the chronic care needs of patients may require that a patient be permanently institutionalized with various services provided on a daily basis—and this is good. But the key questions are, how should we best assess and meet these needs, and should we house these two types of services in different provider settings in view of the far-reaching nature of their differences in orientation and activities?

Our Society's Changing Long-Term Care Needs

As the longevity of the average American increases, bringing about a commensurate increase in the percentage of elderly in our society, the need for long-term care, including nursing home care as well as other types of institutional and noninstitutional long-term care, will continue to grow (HCFA 1987, 1989c; NCHS 1988; Mariano 1989). Almost all forecasts that deal with demographic characteristics, future demand for health care, and the supply required to meet such demand, predict a significant increase in the need for providers of long-term care (Dubay 1989; Scanlon 1988; Harrington, Swan, and Grant 1988; Weissert 1985). As we brace ourselves societally for increased demand for health care due to increases in the elderly population, it becomes more important, in fact critically important, to search for better ways to provide hospital care, physician care, and long-term care. A main theme of this book is that one solution to this dilemma involves recognizing and acting on the fact that hospital discharge is a pivotal entry point to the long-term care delivery system. The actions taken shortly before and after hospital discharge in no small way shape the quality, cost, and effectiveness of our entire health care system.

Since policymakers, health care providers, and researchers have become more concerned about and focused on health care effectiveness, several issues have emerged. Far from insignificant among these issues, particularly as it relates to long-term care, is quality of care. The quality of health care provided after discharge from the hospital has taken on increased importance during the recent past because of the potential deleterious effects of shortened acute stays under Medicare's prospective payment system for hospitals implemented in 1983. This payment system reimburses hospitals not on the basis of total cost, using Medicare's proportion of total days to determine reimbursement—as was previously done. Rather, it reimburses on the basis of prospectively determined prices for the entire inpatient stay by type of patient, providing an incentive for hospitals to discharge patients sooner (Guterman et al. 1988; Sloan, Morrisey, and Valvona 1988a; Weiner et al. 1987).

Hospital stays have shortened considerably (an objective of the new payment system), and there is cause for concern about quality of both hospital and posthospital care (clearly not an objective of the new system) (Neu and Harrison 1988; Moon 1985; Lyles 1986; Shaughnessy and Kramer 1990). Concerns have been voiced that long-term care facilities are not able to properly treat the more intensely ill types of patients now being discharged from acute care hospitals to long-term care settings (Vladeck 1988; Fitzgerald, Moore, and Dittus 1988). These patients, and others with intense medical and skilled care needs who are admitted to nursing homes from the community, are termed *near-acute care* patients in this book. Equally important, strong reservations have been expressed about the quality of care provided in nursing homes in general (IOM 1986).

POLICY CHRONOLOGY

The following several sections provide an overview of the history of nursing home care and the background of how Medicare and Medicaid have influenced the delivery of long-term care. Material from these sections that is essential to understanding the remaining chapters can be found in the Chapter 1 summary if one is not interested in a more detailed discussion of the background issues.

Genesis of Today's Nursing Homes

Although institutional long-term care for the elderly evolved largely out of the political and technological developments of the early and mid–twentieth century, its origins are traceable to the nineteenth century and even colonial practices. Because of the manner in which nursing homes evolved, these institutions today care for patients with chronic care needs and for patients with near-acute care needs.

The institutional precursors of nursing homes, for the most part, housed and maintained the chronically dependent elderly and others but provided few health care services (Dunlop 1979). Noteworthy exceptions, however, included nonprofit general hospitals, which began to appear in substantial numbers throughout the United States in the nineteenth century. The first stages of what we today call administratively necessary days or bed blocking (Safran and Eastwood 1989) were apparent in several communities in the nineteenth century as such hospitals occasionally "found themselves saddled with 'old chronic' patients who developed an acute illness and then could not be discharged to their homes" (Gillick 1989; Rosenberg 1977).

The only formalized system we had for institutional long-term care until the mid–nineteenth century was our system of almshouses and poor farms that were governmentally supported facilities for the destitute poor (Vladeck 1980). The intent was that local governments would care for the "deserving poor" (the retarded, chronically ill, and feeble elderly) in these institutions, rather than providing direct financial assistance. That this system was not the sole institutional supply for long-term care beds is evident in view of the exceptionally long stays at many nonprofit general hospitals. For example, Massachusetts General Hospital had an average stay of 81 days in 1855 (Vogel 1980). Several of the earlier, well-established voluntary hospitals set the pace for other hospitals, however, gradually moving in the direction of shorter-stay institutions. They began to selectively admit acutely ill patients who would likely stay for shorter periods of time, yielding higher turnover and larger numbers of patients, often for teaching or educational purposes. This movement was spurred on by greater technological and scientific advances in medicine in the latter part of the nineteenth and earlier part of the twentieth centuries.

As stays in voluntary general hospitals shortened during the second half of the nineteenth century, to 17–20 days by the turn of the century (Vogel 1980), changes in our institutional long-term care system began to occur. A distinction emerged between the worthy poor (poor out of misfortune), who should have an alternative to the almshouses, and the unworthy poor (poor out of sloth), who now tended to be cared for in almshouses (Gillick 1989). Some private hospitals, chiefly those operated by religious or ethnic groups, established chronic care wards. Other hospitals built freestanding old-age homes (Haber 1983). Many old-age homes appeared that were not affiliated with hospitals. They were basically private charitable homes, at times founded by immigrant groups in the late nineteenth and early twentieth centuries, operating largely along religious and ethnic lines. Such homes developed into the modern voluntary nursing home. In addition to the almshouse or poor farm and the private charitable home or old-age home, a third alternative for long-term care was available. Board and care homes or rest homes were an outgrowth of a practice that saw elderly people residing in private households as paying boarders. Common since colonial times, board and care homes became even more prevalent during the Depression, when people took elderly boarders into their homes to augment their incomes (Vladeck 1980).

Shortly after World War I, mental hospitals emerged as dominant providers of care for the institutionalized elderly. The change from almshouses to mental hospitals was pronounced. Elderly people in mental hospitals outnumbered those in old-age homes and almshouses combined by 1930. This change occurred largely due to state-level statutory changes that appeared around the turn of the century, continuing into the first part of the twentieth century. The laws provided incentives, for example, to reclassify impaired elderly as "psychotic due to arteriosclerosis and senility" and to encourage municipalities to transfer elderly patients to state mental facilities (Grob 1986).

Thus, these institutions—almshouses and poor farms, private charitable homes and old-age homes, board and care homes and rest homes, and mental hospitals—all had their origins prior to the twentieth century. By the early 1930s, the unacceptable conditions in almshouses and a belief that the elderly should not be forced to live in mental institutions contributed to growing support for cash pensions. The Social Security Act of 1935 (c.531, 49 Stat. 620, 42 U.S.C. 301 et seq.) profoundly influenced the evolution of institutional long-term care by supplementing income for the elderly poor through the Old Age Assistance (OAA) program. The federal government matched state contributions under OAA subject to a monthly limit for eligible beneficiaries. States were free to spend as little as they wished and to determine the eligibility criteria for beneficiaries. With this source of supplemental income, eligible individuals were able to choose where to receive care. Many chose to go to private charitable homes or to board and care homes rather than remain wards of the government in undesirable almshouses. In fact, cash assistance payments were prohibited to residents of public facilities in order to eliminate almshouses (Dunlop 1979; Vladeck 1980; Gillick 1989).

Nursing care was selectively added to the service programs of the now-changing successors of private charitable homes and board and care homes, ultimately resulting in more widespread use of the term *nursing home*. Board and care homes, now often operated by private entrepreneurs, began to offer more nursing and personal care services for purposes of gaining a competitive edge (Dunlop 1979; Hawes and Phillips 1986). Private charitable homes for the aged also began to provide health care services. Despite the increased prevalence of nursing homes and the addition of some nursing services, there was a continuing shortage of such facilities in almost all locations. In many communities, general hospitals continued to be used to provide care to persons with chronic illnesses (Dunlop 1979; Vladeck 1980).

Eligibility for, and expanded coverage of, publicly financed nursing home care increased further with the amendments to the Social Security

Act in 1939, 1946, and 1947 (c.666, 53 Stat. 1360; c.951, 60 Stat. 978; and c.510, 61 Stat. 793, respectively). The Social Security Amendments of 1950 (c.809, 64 Stat. 477) ended the exclusion of residents of public facilities from the OAA program. By this time, however, almshouses had disappeared. The new law permitted OAA cash assistance payments to residents of public medical facilities (including public nursing homes). The amendments also allowed for federally matched state and local payments to be made directly to service vendors, a departure from the prior practice of only making direct payments to beneficiaries. States that made such vendor payments were required to establish a program for licensing nursing homes. Thus, the 1950s represented a decade of increasing public influence in the nursing home industry, although public control was characterized by minimal standards, variation in standards, and few active enforcement efforts (Vladeck 1980).

The Hill-Burton Era

After World War II, we systematically and comprehensively undertook to improve our outdated hospitals. The Hospital Survey and Construction Act (the Hill-Burton Act, P.L. 79-725), passed by Congress in 1946, provided $3.7 billion in assistance for health care facility construction and renovation between 1946 and 1971. About $2.6 billion of this went to build or improve acute care hospitals, approximately 10 percent of all hospital construction costs during that period (Lave and Lave 1974). The act was intended to upgrade America's outdated hospitals, especially those in areas with low income or low population density. It helped transform the American health care system, with the hospital as its center (Vladeck 1980).

Hill-Burton ushered in the next phase of decreasing hospital involvement in caring for longer-stay patients with chronic illnesses. Hospitals continued to become more specialized centers for treating acute illnesses and were less willing to use their more expensive settings for patients with chronic conditions. This transformation was largely due to technological and therapeutic advances during World War II, as well as the infusion of dollars to hospitals through Hill-Burton and private health insurance initiated in the 1930s (Dunlop 1979). Nonetheless, this era did not totally eliminate the orientation of selected city and county hospitals to continue to care for patients with chronic diseases.

The effect of Hill-Burton was dramatic in rural America. Before World War II, many rural communities did not have hospitals, relying instead on services provided by one or, at most, a few physicians—and, out of necessity, relying on health care resources in more distant locations to which community residents were required to travel. After the war, however, the practice of medicine had become more technical and hospital-centered. Physicians were even more likely than before to be attracted to communities with hospitals (Koff 1988). At the same time, rural communities were caught up in the country's postwar spirit of renewal and the nation's unprecedented growth. To be ready for the predicted influx of people into rural America, rural communities—even very small ones—wanted to have their own hospitals (personal communication with S. A. Monroe, August 30, 1989).

Hill-Burton helped rural areas achieve this goal by its requirement that states give priority in allocating hospital construction funds to rural communities, where the shortage of beds was the greatest. This requirement was partially premised on the theory that communities with hospitals were more likely to attract physicians and other trained personnel. With the assistance of Hill-Burton funds over a 25-year period, more than 4,400 projects were undertaken to build, expand, or renovate short-term hospitals in communities of 50,000 or fewer people. More than 1,400 new hospitals were built in these communities (Lave and Lave 1974). Nevertheless, the dilemma of how to staff such hospitals (including both physician and nursing staff) existed from the outset. Inadequate consideration was given to whether these smaller communities could support a hospital with adequate demand for inpatient services.

The nursing home industry also benefited from Hill-Burton. As the demand for acute care in hospitals increased, they progressively refocused their resources on acute care rather than chronic care. A serious shortage of nursing home beds for chronic care patients was apparent. As a result, Congress amended Hill-Burton in 1954 to include financing for constructing nursing homes operated in conjunction with a hospital. Funded by Hill-Burton, these new nursing homes were under the jurisdiction of the Public Health Service. Because of this, their structural design, construction, staffing patterns, and related characteristics were influenced by hospital-like standards. Although proprietary nursing homes were originally excluded from Hill-Burton funding, lobbying by the American Nursing Home Association led to authorization for Small Business Administration loans in 1956 and Federal Housing Administration loan insurance for capital expenditures for proprietary facilities in 1959 (Dunlop 1979; Vladeck 1980; Hawes and Phillips 1986; Gillick 1989).

The Kerr-Mills Approach

The Kerr-Mills bill, passed by Congress in 1960 (P.L. 83-788), increased vendor payments for nursing homes, under the Medical Assistance for the Aged (MAA) program. This was a forerunner of today's Medicaid program, providing medical assistance for the low-income aged. States were permitted to define medical indigency separately from the need for income assistance, allowing elderly people with incomes too high for OAA payments to qualify for direct vendor payments for medical care (including nursing home care) if the cost of care were judged to be beyond their means (Dunlop 1979).

By 1966, all but three states had established an MAA program of some sort. However, Kerr-Mills left program design to individual states, resulting in considerable interstate variation. Two states never appropriated funds for their MAA programs, and only five states established programs that were considered comprehensive. Nevertheless, by 1965 MAA had paid for the care of 300,000 nursing home residents, increasing government outlays for nursing home care nearly tenfold since Kerr-Mills was enacted (Vladeck 1980; IOM 1986).

The Big Bang: Medicare and Medicaid

No single event in our country's history impacted our health care system as substantially and pervasively as the passage of the Social Security Act Amendments of 1965 (P.L. 89-97), which established the Medicare and Medicaid programs. These programs would ultimately result in radically increased public financing for the elderly, disabled, and poor. They would also dramatically influence health policy in both the public and private sectors during the next several decades.

With respect to nursing home care, the original intent under Medicare was that the Medicare nursing home benefit should save money that would have otherwise been spent on extended hospital care. The law limited Medicare payments to 100 days of convalescent care in an extended care facility (ECF) after at least 3 days of hospitalization (the 3-day prior hospitalization requirement persists today, despite a brief period when it was eliminated). ECFs were originally required to meet relatively stringent standards for certification as Medicare providers (Hawes and Phillips 1986).

The Medicaid program extended the Kerr-Mills approach, providing medical coverage to federal welfare recipients and to medically indigent of all ages. Under Medicaid, skilled nursing home (SNH) care was a mandated service. Certification criteria for SNHs were originally left to individual states; mandatory federal criteria were not established until several years later (Dunlop 1979). However, interim guidelines called for Medicaid SNHs to meet essentially the same standards as Medicare ECFs (Vladeck 1980).

With the massive influx of federal financing under Medicare, it became apparent that the objective of saving Medicare dollars by replacing hospital care with less expensive nursing home care would probably not become a reality. Considerably more inpatient care was being provided with Medicare financing than had been estimated. Fearing an inadequate supply of certified hospitals to care for Medicare patients, the Bureau of Health Insurance (BHI) in the Social Security Administration (SSA) determined that hospitals—and by extension, nursing homes—that were in "substantial compliance" with certification requirements, and that demonstrated an intent to improve, could be certified for reimbursement for care provided to Medicare beneficiaries. About 6,000 of the nation's 13,000 nursing homes at that time applied for Medicare ECF certification. Of these, 740 fully complied, and 3,200 others were found to be in substantial compliance (Vladeck 1980).

The 1967 Moss amendments to the Social Security Act (P.L. 90-248) made federal Medicaid nursing home guidelines more stringent. They resulted from the work of the Subcommittee on Long-Term Care of the Senate's Special Committee on Aging chaired by Senator Frank Moss of Utah. The intent was to address inadequate conditions in nursing homes including poorly trained, unknowledgeable administrators, professional staff shortages, and fire and safety problems. Several of the regulations subsequently issued to implement the amendments fell short of the subcommittee's intent, especially those dealing with better nursing supervision in nursing homes. Even so, the nursing home industry proposed a new type of nursing home, the intermediate care facility (ICF), for patients requiring less intense nursing home care. The ICF was created by the 1967 Miller amendment to the Social Security Act. It was accepted by Congress with little opposition, at least in part because so few nursing homes were able to meet either the Medicare standards for ECFs or the less stringent Medicaid SNH regulations. Many states merely reclassified facilities (as ICFs) that could not meet the Moss amendment's staffing and "life safety code" requirements. ICFs were not considered medical facilities and were originally eligible for payments only under the OAA program of the Social Security Act. They were brought under Medicaid in 1971 by P.L. 92-223 (Vladeck 1980; Dunlop 1979).

To control escalating costs resulting from the substantial compliance policy, the Bureau of Health Insurance issued Intermediary Letter 371 in April 1969. The letter listed services that a facility had to offer if it wished to provide extended care and defined "skilled nursing" more narrowly. It required that recipients have "rehabilitation potential" (Dunlop 1979). The letter also made it clear that fiscal intermediaries that administered the Medicare reimbursement program should apply requirements stringently. The result was a dramatic increase in claims denials, from 1.5 percent of claims in 1968 to 8.2 percent in 1970. Many of the denials were made retroactively. A number of nursing homes were unable to collect payments from patients (or their families or estates) after such denials. As a result, more than 500 facilities dropped their Medicare certification during the period following issuance of Intermediary Letter 371. Medicare, which had paid more than 1 million nursing home claims in 1968, paid for less than 400,000 in 1972, reducing nursing home outlays by more than half (Vladeck 1980).

The 1972 Amendments to the Social Security Act (P.L. 92-603), enacted in October 1972, consolidated Medicare ECFs and Medicaid SNHs, terming them "skilled nursing facilities" (SNFs). The Department of Health, Education, and Welfare (HEW) was instructed to develop a single set of certification standards for such facilities. To reduce retroactive claim denials, "presumptive eligibility" for SNF admission was created for particular diagnoses. The law also provided for full federal funding of state certification and enforcement activities. It required state Medicaid reimbursement for both SNFs and ICFs to be made on a "reasonable cost-related basis." Watergate delayed full implementation of these amendments, so that regulations to implement the SNF certification standards and cost-related reimbursement did not go into effect until mid-1974 and early 1978, respectively (Dunlop 1979; Vladeck 1980).

Where We Are Today

In sum, the various and sundry predecessors of nursing homes prior to 1930 were hewn and shaped by a series of public policy initiatives between the 1930s and early 1970s to form the basis for the nursing home industry as we know it today. Noteworthy was the relative absence of physician involvement in the evolution of the nursing home industry, a phenomenon that accounts for the minimal involvement of physicians in the field today. This is reinforced by the relatively low Medicare and Medicaid reimbursement for physician care of nursing home patients.

By the late 1960s and early 1970s, although public policy had greatly increased the supply of nursing homes, concerns continued to grow about access to and adequacy of nursing home care. This contributed to the concerns about quality of care and quality of life in nursing homes that persist today. Many communities, especially rural communities, still had a paucity of nursing homes owing to the inability of the industry to meet federal certification standards. Yet, many rural communities, in large part due to Hill-Burton, had community hospitals that were often underoccupied. A classification system for different types of long-term care and acute care was ensconced as part of the Medicare program. Certification standards were different for hospital, SNF, and ICF patients. Although SNF beds could be certified as ICF beds, hospital beds could not be certified as either SNF or ICF beds.

Several critical policy initiatives that occurred after the mid-1970s are presented in ensuing chapters. The intent in this chapter has been to present an overview of selected topics that set the stage for what would ultimately prove to be an effective program for providing near-acute long-term care in hospital beds.

OBJECTIVES OF THIS BOOK

The purpose of this book is twofold. First, it is intended to trace the rather unusual, but highly informative, evolution of hospital swing beds (i.e., hospital beds used for both acute and long-term care). Second, it is aimed at isolating what we have learned from this evolutionary process in order to improve the cost effectiveness with which we provide long-term care in the United States, particularly for near-acute care patients.

The following five chapters which make up Part II, document the manner in which the swing-bed story unfolded in the 1970s and the 1980s. While the policy history of swing beds is unusual, it will become clear that the success of the swing-bed approach did not occur by happenstance. Rather, as providers experimented with ways to provide swing-bed care, it became apparent that critical ingredients of long-term care that were often missing in other settings were beginning to occur in swing-bed settings. Greater coordination of a patient's care needs at the interface between acute care and long-term care began to occur, physician involvement in long-term care was more pronounced, skilled nursing care and certain types of rehabilitation care were more available, patients more frequently developed the attitude that they truly would recover from strokes or serious injuries, and, perhaps above all, different providers of care exchanged greater amounts of information necessary in helping the patient through various transitions from one level of care to another.

It took a considerable amount of time for us to realize that these types of ingredients were among the dominant reasons for the success of the swing-bed program. It appears to be taking us even longer to ascertain just how to transport them to other settings. In this regard, this book is not intended to be a diatribe against nursing homes or other providers of long-term care. Far from it. Rather, in view of the many thousands of nursing homes we have in our country and the absolutely critical role they play in our health care system, this book issues a challenge to nursing homes and other providers of long-term care. What is being done in swing-bed hospitals can be done in other long-term care environments. It is critical that we understand the reasons for superior care and transport these to other settings. Meeting this challenge is not straightforward. The precise manner in which the essential ingredients of care, especially coordination between and among different types of providers, can be implemented and sustained in other long-term care settings is complex, but possible to accomplish.

These types of issues are covered in more depth in Part III (Chapters 7 and 8), where the basic facts of the swing-bed program presented in Part II are augmented by additional information from other relevant long-term care settings and topic areas. The main theme in Part III is that near-acute care can be significantly enhanced in the United States, and that we have a reasonably strong information base which we might use to begin the improvement process through research, demonstrations, and policy initiatives.

Returning to the substance of the first two sections of this chapter, throughout the 1970s, 1980s, and even into the 1990s, as a society, we have not adequately addressed several issues in providing near-acute care. Many patients who should be rehabilitated are not, for a variety of different reasons. To provide the crucial types of near-acute care services necessary for a given patient, we must determine ways to better integrate services that are currently provided in a variety of different settings, such as hospital, nursing home, outpatient, and in-home settings. Professionals in the health care field, including skilled nurses, physicians, rehabilitation therapists, social workers, and home health care providers, must better coordinate the manner in which they provide services and exchange information about patients. Patient status must be monitored relative to expected goals and prognoses initially established in one provider setting, but requiring follow-through in other settings.

In the early 1970s, care coordination and integration was even less adequate than at the present time. Many questioned the quality of nursing home care. Ways to lessen access barriers for certain types of patients in need of long-term care and ways to satisfy the steadily increasing demand for nursing home care were not readily apparent. Yet, it was apparent in the early 1970s that we had extra hospital beds in many communities. The problem of too few nursing home beds and too many hospitals beds was pronounced in rural communities. The history of what happened at this point, beginning with a small experimental program in rural Utah, is presented in the next several chapters.

CHAPTER 1 SUMMARY

Substantial numbers of individuals in the United States are admitted to and retained in nursing homes out of a misguided sense of concern that such individuals cannot regain the capacity to function independently. Many people—just how many is unknown—are discharged from hospitals to nursing homes without adequate assessment of their rehabilitation potential and the health care needed to fully rehabilitate them. Some are unnecessarily retained in nursing homes for the rest of their lives.

That hospital discharge is a key entry point to our long-term care system is often overlooked. Long-term care patients whose needs are close to those of hospital or acute care patients, termed *near-acute care* patients in this book, are not adequately distinguished from longer-term chronic care patients by our regulatory and reimbursement systems, or by our health care providers, communities, and practices. This is in part due to inadequate recognition of the implications of the difference between rehabilitative/restorative care and maintenance/chronic care. We have a ponderous financing system and an accompanying organizational and regulatory structure in place that makes it difficult to change long-term care so that elderly patients with rehabilitation potential can be cost-effectively rehabilitated in our society. As long-term care needs, especially for the elderly, are changing and intensifying at a fairly rapid rate, issues involving the quality of long-term care have become critical to health policymakers.

Since nursing homes are now our dominant providers of publicly financed long-term care, the historical paths we took to reach the circumstances that surround today's nursing homes are informative in analyzing potential solutions to our long-term care problems. By the mid-1800s, the primary providers of institutional long-term care in the United States were local government–sponsored almshouses for the destitute poor, and voluntary general hospitals that cared for the chronically ill as well as the acutely ill. Less formally, private individuals sometimes took into their homes, termed rest homes, elderly people who were moderately dependent and able to pay for board and rest care. As the nineteenth century came to a close, the unacceptable conditions in almshouses, and a trend that saw voluntary hospitals caring for fewer chronically ill patients, led to an increase in private charitable homes for the aged that were initially sponsored by religious and ethnic groups. An increase in mental hospitals as significant providers of institutional long-term care occurred in the first part of the twentieth century.

The Old Age Assistance (OAA) Act of 1935, by virtue of providing cash pensions to needy elderly, who could use such funds to defer the costs of nonpublic (i.e., excluding almshouses) institutional long-term care, substantially changed the direction of long-term care in the United States. As a result of this law, more health care, especially nursing care, was provided in facilities that were now becoming more like today's nursing homes. The old-age or private charitable homes proved to be the forerunners of today's voluntary nursing homes, while the rest homes or board and care homes emerged as the forerunners of today's proprietary nursing homes. Other amendments to the Social Security Act in the 1930s, 1940s, and 1950s both strengthened public influence in the nursing home industry and permitted government payments to be made directly to service providers rather than exclusively to beneficiaries.

The Hill-Burton Act in the mid-1940s provided substantial financial assistance for hospitals to focus more exclusively on acute illnesses and less on chronic care, moving hospitals further from the provision of institutional long-term care. During the 1940s, 1950s, and 1960s, the Hill-Burton program served as a catalyst both to reorient the hospital industry and to build large numbers of new hospitals, especially in rural communities, throughout the United States. During this period, demand for institutional long-term care continued to go unmet in many communities in the United States, despite the availability of Hill-Burton funds to finance capital expansion in the nursing home field as well as the hospital field.

In 1960, the Medical Assistance for the Aged Act (Kerr-Mills) was enacted. It proved to be a precursor of today's Medicaid program, focusing on medical assistance for the low-income aged. It revised the Old Age Assistance program approach, permitting direct vendor payments for medical care, including nursing home care, for elderly with incomes above the OAA limits. The Kerr-Mills approach was characterized by considerable interstate variation. However, it served to significantly increase government outlays for, and involvement in, the nursing home field.

Public sector influence of the health care system was strengthened with the enactment of the Medicare and Medicaid programs in 1965. The Medicare nursing home benefit was initially intended to save money that would have otherwise been spent on extended hospital care. The Medicare extended care facility (ECF) was targeted on this objective. Medicaid skilled nursing homes (SNHs) were mandated, with Medicaid certification criteria originally left to individual states. Certification criteria were eventually made uniform for ECFs and SNHs, subsequently called skilled nursing facilities (SNFs). Medicaid intermediate care facilities (ICFs) were established to provide institutional long-term care that did not require significant amounts of skilled nursing care. As we continued to wrestle with our approach to institutional long-term care in the late 1960s and early 1970s, our public programs resulted in an incentive structure that brought about an increase in the number of certified facilities providing skilled nursing care in the late 1960s, followed by a decrease in the number of such facilities by the early 1970s. Throughout the evolutionary period for today's nursing homes, conspicuously absent was comprehensive and substantive input from the physician community on the essential aspects of long-term care from the perspective of medical care.

By the early 1970s, concerns about the quality of nursing home care, inadequate access to nursing home care, and how to meet the demand for nursing home care were of considerable consequence. At the same time, health planners recognized that we had built too many hospital beds. The dilemma of an inadequate supply of institutional long-term care providers and too many hospital beds was particularly manifest in rural communities throughout the United States. The stage was set for a small program in rural Utah that would ultimately point the way to at least one solution to this dilemma.

PART II

The Evolution of
Hospital Swing Beds

CHAPTER 2

The Beginning of Swing Beds:
The Utah Experiment

PURPOSES SERVED BY THE SWING-BED APPROACH

The Swing-Bed Idea

In early October 1969, four state officials were traveling by car between the towns of Moab and Monticello in eastern Utah. They were in the process of surveying hospitals for Medicare certification. In some ways, rural Utah was no different from many other rural areas throughout the country. It was characterized by a number of relatively new hospitals whose construction, renovation, or both had been financed by the Hill-Burton program. The hospitals were surveyed annually in order to be certified as complying with Medicare standards necessary to receive reimbursement for care provided to Medicare patients.

As was the case nationally, residents of rural Utah benefited considerably from the greater access to acute care and medical care afforded under Hill-Burton. Nonetheless, as is the case today, the demand for acute care was uneven and episodic in small rural communities throughout the country. Rural hospitals often lack the financial advantages that accrue from economies of scale and various types of shared service arrangements more commonplace in metropolitan areas. The significant increases in demand for inpatient hospital care that had been forecast during the Hill-Burton era, and even more recently since the inception of Medicare and Medicaid, never materialized in rural areas as strongly as some had forecast. Consequently, rural hospitals were in the early 1970s, and are today, frequently unstable and faced with possible closure. Medicare- and Medicaid-certified nursing homes, by contrast, have typically been characterized by high occupancy rates and by patient waiting lists in many rural communities.

As the surveyors discussed what could be done to assist the community of Moab in preserving its hospital as both a source of acute care and a crucial cog in the economy of the small community, they talked about the relatively strong unmet need for nursing home care for chronically ill patients. Elderly residents of Moab were being transported considerable distances to metropolitan nursing homes or to nursing homes in other rural communities far from their families and home support systems. The question arose that ultimately gave birth to the swing-bed program: Why not provide nursing home care in empty hospital beds in this particular community? Can we not simply use these beds for both hospital care and nursing home care? Beyond this, should we not consider this option in other places in rural Utah in view of the excess of hospital beds and the shortage of nursing home beds in rural communities?

Present in the car was a physician named Bruce Walter, the director of Medicare services in Utah at that time and later the director of the Utah State Division of Health. It was Bruce Walter who first proposed the swing-bed concept and initially implemented it. He was an intense individual—persistent, dedicated, even pugnacious, and not likely to give up on an idea that he thought had merit. In fact, given the crusader that he was, he was the right person at the right time, since it would not prove easy to convince either hospital staff or government officials that the merits of his idea of "swinging" hospital beds between acute and long-term care outweighed its disadvantages.

Impediments and Rationale

People familiar with rural health care at that time were aware that significant progress had been made in the previous two decades in reducing discrepancies between rural and urban communities in terms of access to health care services. Yet, they also knew that health care in many rural areas was handicapped by a shortage of qualified personnel and a lack of comprehensive services—problems that persist today (Ermann 1990; U.S. Congress OTA 1990). Physicians can feel isolated in rural areas where a community often depends on but one or a few physicians. A lack of staff and technological resources makes rural practice difficult for physicians. The distance rural residents sometimes have to travel to obtain ambulatory care—to say nothing of both acute care and long-term care—was recognized as more than a simple matter of inconvenience. Access to an acute care hospital in an emergency can represent the difference between long-term disability and complete recovery, between high and low cost of care, or even between life and death under certain circumstances.

Bruce Walter and others recognized that a shortage of adequate nursing home care in rural communities results in placing long-term care patients in distant nursing homes and detracts from the ability of family and friends to visit. Consequently, it affects the quality of life for elderly residents in an institutional setting. Such problems can be exacerbated by the long stays often associated with nursing home care.

Therefore, in response to the dilemma of excess hospital beds and a paucity of Medicare- and Medicaid-certified nursing home beds in rural communities, the swing-bed concept was born in rural Utah in 1969. It would be several years, however, before Bruce Walter would succeed in putting it in place in even a few rural hospitals in his state.

One of the hurdles facing the program arose from concerns about excess supply. These concerns gave birth to the health planning movement that flourished in the United States in the 1970s. Having its voluntary roots in the state health planning agencies encouraged under the Hill-Burton program begun in 1946 and its more formal inception beginning with the establishment of Regional Medical Programs and Comprehensive Health Planning Agencies in 1966, this movement led to the National Health Planning and Resources Development Act of 1974 (P.L. 93-641), which created 213 health systems agencies throughout the United States. These agencies were directed to actively influence grants, loans, and reimbursement for health care institutions in their respective health services areas (Koff 1988; Hyman 1977). Most health planners and many health policymakers had agreed by the early 1970s that we had too many hospital beds in the United States. Despite the best of intentions under Hill-Burton, we were now overbedded with acute care hospital beds, even with the increased utilization resulting from the Medicare and Medicaid programs. Concerns about hospital costs and excess beds continued to increase throughout the 1970s and 1980s. It was at about this time, roughly five years after the inception of Medicare and Medicaid, that these concerns established a strong foothold in the health policy environment.

The potential value of the swing-bed approach was initially preempted by a broader policy question: Why should we bother keeping these rural hospitals open? Clearly they were contributing to our surplus bed capacity. Are not efforts to maintain such beds unnecessarily increasing costs? Yet, an analysis of this issue showed that if we closed 20 percent of all rural hospitals, we would reduce total hospital costs in the

United States by only 3.4 percent, an amount substantially below the annual inflation rate for hospital costs (Shaughnessy 1978).

On the other hand, the reasons for considering the swing-bed approach were persuasive (Shaughnessy 1984). The concept was premised on several assumptions about the health care delivery system in rural areas:

1. An unmet demand for institutional long-term care exists in many rural communities, especially, as would later be demonstrated in states outside Utah, for near-acute care that requires more intense medical and skilled nursing services than provided in typical rural nursing homes.
2. Surplus staff capacity is present in a number of underoccupied rural hospitals.
3. Providing adequate long-term care is possible in a hospital setting if staff members are sufficiently acquainted with the administrative and patient-level aspects of providing such care.
4. Providing long-term care in existing rural hospitals is potentially more cost-effective than other alternatives in meeting the demand for institutional long-term care in rural communities.
5. Benefits can accrue to long-term care patients, their families, and friends by providing care in the patient's home community rather than more distant locations.
6. Using the resources of rural hospitals for long-term care can contribute to the preservation of small community hospitals, resulting in the continued availability of acute care, diversifying the service program of rural hospitals, and maintaining such hospitals as vital parts of the economy of rural communities.

Although not included in the original tenets of the swing-bed approach, the issue of near-acute versus chronic care for long-term care patients would also become a pivotal topic in the late 1970s and the 1980s. Initially, the relative paucity of nursing home beds in rural communities led to the seemingly obvious conclusion that a uniform shortage of all types of nursing home care existed in rural areas. However, as experience was gained in locations outside Utah, it became more apparent that the most significant need was for near-acute long-term care in these communities. As originally conceived, however, the Utah project was designed to encourage swing-bed hospitals to provide both chronic and near-acute care in hospital swing beds.

THE FIRST SWING-BED PROGRAM:
THE UTAH COST-IMPROVEMENT PROJECT

The Early Struggle

In October 1969, upon his return to Salt Lake City, Bruce Walter wrote a letter to Wilburn Smith at the regional Medicare office in Denver, describing his idea that long-term care patients could be cared for in acute care hospital beds at long-term care reimbursement rates. Smith considered the idea worthwhile and supported it within the Denver regional office. He suggested that the staff at Medicare headquarters in Baltimore consider it seriously.

Rumor has it that the several rounds of negotiations that took place to get the Utah swing-bed experiment off the ground were frequently more than a little tense. The impediments that caused the rather rocky start were understandable and, to everyone's credit, ultimately overcome. The Medicare program was still young, feeling its way along in dealing with innovation, both administratively and bureaucratically. The organizational structure that many of us consider almost synonymous with Medicare and Medicaid, the Health Care Financing Administration (HCFA), was still several years away from its formal inception. In fact, it was not until the Department of Health, Education, and Welfare was reorganized in 1977 that HCFA came into being as an organizational entity.

The swing-bed idea being proposed was a variation on a theme in practice before the advent of Medicare and Medicaid in 1965. As discussed in the first chapter, it was not unusual for hospitals, especially prior to or during the early stages of the Hill-Burton era, to care for both acute and long-term care patients, reducing long-term care patients' payment rates as considered appropriate by the hospital's administration. Medicare and Medicaid regulations for long-term care facilities, however, restricted the flexibility of acute care hospitals to provide long-term care. These new public insurance programs encouraged institutional alternatives to the hospitals for long-term care patients. The extended care facility (ECF) was viewed as an appropriate setting especially for aged patients discharged from acute care in general hospitals (Moroney and Kurtz 1975). While the ECF, along with Medicaid skilled nursing homes (SNHs), ultimately evolved into the skilled nursing facility (SNF), it was regarded as the institution of choice for posthospital skilled nursing and rehabilitative care, as distinct from more prolonged chronic care.

With this option available, why bother with swing beds? Why not simply convert hospital beds to ECF beds? The answer to this question rested with the rigidity of the new Medicare regulations for nursing homes. To be reimbursed for the provision of skilled nursing care under Medicare, a nursing home had to be certified, demonstrating that the facility meets a variety of requirements. For hospitals to provide long-term care, the certification requirements specified that the hospital should provide a physically distinct part (e.g., building, wing, corridor) exclusively for the provision of long-term care. The hospital was also required to establish and maintain separate financial records for its skilled nursing unit and to provide specialized services such as physical therapy, social services, and patient activities. These long-term care beds could not be used for acute care, nor could acute care beds be used for long-term care under the Medicare rules.

As also mentioned in Chapter 1, the consolidation of Medicare ECFs and Medicaid SNHs into a new category of certified nursing home, SNFs, further reduced the supply of available nursing homes (U.S. Congress, Senate 1974). The net effect of the new law was that Medicare and Medicaid facilities had greater difficulty in meeting the certification standards. Most Medicare ECFs had been certified only by virtue of substantial compliance. Due to Intermediary Letter 371, many were also encountering frequent retroactive claims denials. Medicaid SNHs that previously met relatively minimal state standards had further to go to comply with the new regulatory standards.

Since demand for acute care services in rural areas remained unchanged relative to the oversupply of acute care beds, and since Medicare- and Medicaid-certified nursing home beds were now in even greater demand in such communities, the policy climate was conducive to supporting the swing-bed concept. Bruce Walter struggled to promote the idea through several meetings in Baltimore and Washington. In February 1970 and September 1972, he made presentations to the Subcommittee on Long-Term Care of the Special Senate Committee on Aging chaired by Senator Frank Moss of Utah. Valid questions, such as how to structure reimbursement and why the Medicare hospital-based ECF alternative was not acceptable, were raised and reraised on various occasions. Requirements that should be imposed on hospitals that might participate in such a program were discussed. Should not hospitals that were going to provide nursing home care also have to satisfy all certification standards and requirements that nursing homes are required to meet? On the other hand, if some sort of an experimental program were to be launched, with Medicare possibly waiving standard reimbursement or certification policies, what guarantees would there be that hospitals would even participate?

One of the meetings held during the negotiation phase was noteworthy: the "Great Table" meeting (personal communication with Bruce

Walter, August 15, 1989). This gathering was convened in April 1972, largely through the efforts of Frank Moss, to present the supporting evidence on swing beds to Tom Tierney (Medicare's first director) and other ranking Medicare officials. Bruce Walter had also found a willing listener in Jerry Scheinbeck, head of Medicare's Survey Certification Section in Baltimore, who was instrumental in moving the idea ahead. In addition, Walter asked Clarence Wonnackott, a former American Hospital Association president, to help sway Tierney.

"When we entered the conference room, we encountered the longest table I had ever seen," Walter recalled. The table was so large that some jokingly speculated that the conference room in the Social Security Administration (SSA) building had been built around it. "Tom Tierney and the other Medicare people sat at one end of the table, and Charles Maxwell and I sat all the way at the other end, with our projector and screen. I was struck by the symbolism." Walter and Maxwell successfully bridged the abyss, however. The meeting ended with Tierney saying, "We'll see what we can do." Walter optimistically took this response as close to yes and doggedly pursued the idea.

The First Success: An Experimental Program

To the credit of Bruce Walter, Wilburn Smith, Jerry Scheinbeck, and others who had persisted for several years, a contract ensued shortly thereafter that permitted a handful of rural hospitals to see what they could do with the swing-bed idea. Termed the Utah Cost Improvement Project (UCIP), the Utah swing-bed experiment began in January 1973. The project was the product of an extended period of communication and negotiation between the Utah State Division of Health and SSA. It was funded as a three-year experiment under Sections 402 and 222(b) of the Social Security amendments of 1967 and 1972, respectively. Section 402 involved incentive reimbursement and was influential in determining the original orientation of UCIP as a reimbursement project, as opposed to a purely service-oriented project. The project was twice extended and continued until the national swing-bed program went into effect in the early 1980s. Section 222(b) provided the demonstration authority for the project.

Formally, the administrative vehicle for the UCIP was a contract between the Program Experimentation Branch in the Bureau of Health Insurance, SSA, and the Utah State Division of Health, the administering agency for the demonstration. When the Department of Health, Education, and Welfare was reorganized in 1977, the Office of Demonstrations and Evaluations of HCFA assumed administration of the Utah project.

The Medicare fiscal intermediary in Utah, Blue Cross, was responsible for Medicare reimbursement for long-term care to participating UCIP hospitals. The Utah Medicaid program also participated in the experiment. Many long-term care patients paid out of pocket for care received in swing beds. Medicare and Medicaid were the only third party payers who participated in the experiment. Medicare reimbursed for only skilled nursing care, whereas Medicaid reimbursed for skilled nursing, intermediate, and personal care.

By definition, the skilled nursing care patient required the most intense level of long-term care, the level closest to traditional inpatient acute care. The skilled nursing care patient is one whose acute care needs have been met, but, according to regulations in effect at the time of UCIP, usually required extended nursing care under the supervision of both physician and professional registered nursing personnel. A skilled nursing facility was required to have a transfer agreement with an acute care hospital to promptly provide acute care services when necessary.

The other two levels of care were covered by Medicaid only. Intermediate care patients under UCIP generally required supportive nursing care, often provided by a licensed practical nurse rather than a registered professional nurse. Care at the intermediate level is beyond that available through a purely residential or domiciliary care program, and as a practical matter, is usually available only in institutional settings. Personal care, as it pertained to Utah Medicaid during 1973 through 1975, was basically a second level of intermediate care not requiring as much nursing care as the first level just described.

Hospitals participating in the UCIP experiment were not required to satisfy all Medicare and Medicaid certification standards for long-term care. Although some of the standards for hospitals and skilled nursing facilities overlapped, swing-bed hospitals were not required to meet the standards relating to rehabilitation services (physical, speech, and occupational therapy), rehabilitative nursing, dental services, social services, and patient activity space, among others. Analogously, Medicaid regulations for intermediate and personal care in Utah that were not already embodied in the acute care regulations were waived for the experimental hospitals.

A formula for reimbursing project hospitals for the delivery of long-term care was established. Medicare covered only skilled nursing care and paid the Medicaid skilled per diem under the Utah experiment. However, Medicare reimbursement under UCIP was more complicated than Medicaid since it was related to acute care reimbursement and to a financial incentive payment that was provided to each hospital after Medicare cost reports had been audited and certain incremental costs calculated and approved. The costs of ancillary services (e.g., laboratory and x-ray) for swing-bed patients were paid through the normal Medicare reimbursement mechanism for ancillary services.

These two factors—waivers of Medicare conditions of participation for long-term care and the new reimbursement mechanism, combined with the use of acute care beds to provide both long-term care and acute care—constituted the key elements that defined the experimental nature of the swing-bed project in Utah.

The eligibility criteria for participating hospitals required that each hospital have fewer than 100 beds and less than 60 percent occupancy for the three years prior to the project's implementation. In the original proposal submitted by the Utah State Division of Health to SSA, 12 rural hospitals were identified as meeting the eligibility criteria and willing to participate in the project.

The initial orientation to the project involved a workshop conducted by the State Division of Health on June 1, 1973, for hospital administrators, business office personnel, and directors of nursing. Additional information was provided through written guidelines, ranging from memos sent to hospitals during the first six months of the project to a more comprehensive set of guidelines developed during the third quarter of 1973. A series of brochures describing the project to physicians, nurses, and patients was published in 1974, with a monthly newsletter discussing UCIP progress, activities, and problems, initiated for participating hospitals beginning in late 1974. Continuing education under UCIP was provided through a course in health facilities administration and regional nursing workshops. Meetings of the Utah Small Hospital Association provided opportunities to discuss problems and questions related to the experiment. The program was run under the overall guidance of Bruce Walter. Kent Aland, chief of the Program Development Division of the Bureau of Medical Care Services, served as project director, and R. Donald West, a member of the staff in the Bureau of Medical Care Services, was project coordinator on UCIP.

As the program was implemented in the earlier hospitals that admitted long-term care patients to hospital swing beds, it was apparent that a number of problems would have to be ironed out. Yet, it also appeared that the program would meet the community need for long-term care. As patients were admitted to long-term care from acute care, many of them, along with their families, preferred to be in their community hospital rather than in a nursing home, especially a distant nursing home.

Patients requiring near-acute care after myocardial infarctions and hip fractures, or those with postsurgical recovery needs, were admitted to long-term care from acute care. For many such patients, Medicare was the primary payer. However, a number of patients required chronic care and maintenance care in the general areas of incontinence, cognitive impairments, and functional disabilities relating to ambulating, eating, dressing, and toileting. For such patients, Medicaid and private pay (i.e., not Medicare) were the primary sources of payment. In all, however, both patient and patient families appeared to welcome the swing-bed program in their communities when the need for admission to long-term care arose. The existence of the program was promulgated largely by word of mouth in the various communities, so that it took a reasonable length of time for many residents of the rural communities to even become aware that such a program was in place in their community hospitals.

The apparent value of the program seemed to overcome a number of start-up difficulties. For example, more than one-third of the hospital administrators would subsequently express some negativism about the methods used by the State Division of Health to enlist hospital participation in the demonstration. Due to the time constraints associated with the final SSA contract, staff members at the Division of Health attempted to proceed expeditiously in urging hospitals to participate in the demonstration. Several hospital administrators complained that they felt unduly pressured by the Division of Health, which they contended used its leverage in the areas of hospital licensure, certification, and reimbursement to coerce selected hospitals to participate. In view of the relatively positive response of such administrators to the swing-bed program in general, however, the approach taken by the State Division of Health did not appear to be detrimental and, under the circumstances, may have been necessary.

At the hospital level, the decision of whether to move a patient from one room to another when discharged from acute care and admitted to long-term care was an important issue that hospital staff dealt with separately in each individual hospital. The acclimation of the staff necessary to satisfy a patient's long-term care needs, especially emotional needs and functional support needs over an extended period, was something that would necessarily take time. Acquainting the patient and patient's family with the difference between acute care and long-term care, in view of the fact that long-term care was being provided in a hospital setting, was important. The paperwork associated with Medicare and Medicaid billing and reimbursement imposed a number of difficulties and procedural hurdles that took time to work through. As we will see in the remainder of this chapter, however, the program would persist, largely because of its value to residents and rural communities.

In the months just before and after the initiation of UCIP, opposition to the swing-bed program came from several quarters. The individualism that has often characterized the staff of many rural hospitals throughout the country was certainly not an asset to the swing-bed approach in its early days. This individualism, which exists out of necessity and often serves such facilities well, saw the federal intervention that would accompany Medicare reimbursement for this new concept as something both foreign and unwelcome. The idea that Medicare would pay hospitals at nursing home payment rates was not well received. Both Bruce Walter and the "foreigners" from Washington/Baltimore were trying to explain to hospital staff that the hospital already exists to provide acute care, and that they need not build nor maintain beds or staff to provide additional long-term care (unless the hospital were to go into the long-term care business in a big way). Therefore, hospitals should be paid on the basis of the incremental cost of providing long-term care in an already existing and staffed physical plant. To many hospital administrators this new reimbursement approach just did not make sense.

The relatively new Medicare program was stumbling its way along, with all its new rules and regulations. It was viewed by many health care providers as the ultimate bureaucratic intruder, taking on an obstreperous personality of its own, wanting more and more control simply because it was starting to pay for a reasonably hefty minority of the patient care costs in hospitals. The new intruder was disliked—except for the fact that it did pay for a lot of hospital care. The feeling was somewhat mutual. Why, asked some Medicare officials, should we try to keep these little inefficient hospitals open if they don't want our help and are underoccupied anyway?

Opposition would also come from another sector in the health care field. Nursing home professionals voiced concerns that the hospitals' use of acute care beds for long-term care would cut into their business, reducing nursing home admissions and ultimately eroding their revenue base. Proponents of the nursing home industry voiced the reasonably logical caution that hospital staff are typically not trained to provide long-term care, know very little about it, and would probably do a poor job. Besides, it was likely that hospital staff would not be receptive to caring for nursing home patients in hospital beds. After all, they were trained hospital professionals, who were not likely to be keen about the idea that their hospital would become more like a nursing home.

In addition to substituting for nursing home care in either rural communities or more distant urban areas, other types of substitution were possible. While these were not considered until several years after the Utah swing-bed demonstration had been put in place, they were viable alternatives. Perhaps patients would spend less time (i.e., fewer days) in acute care before being discharged to long-term care. Maybe potential long-term care patients who should have been receiving institutional care were receiving (possibly inappropriate) ambulatory or outpatient care. Swing-bed long-term care might therefore substitute for acute care or physician/outpatient care. Of course, the possibility also existed that some community residents in need of institutional long-term care were receiving no care at all.

In one way or another, these concerns and issues were all reasonable. Each of them ultimately had to be addressed in the process of examining the viability of the swing-bed approach in the 1970s.

RESULTS FROM THE UTAH EXPERIMENT

The Evaluation Study

In view of several important policy questions regarding the viability and cost effectiveness of swing beds raised in the negotiation stages of the UCIP, and in view of the program's potential value if implemented nationally, the Evaluative Studies Branch at SSA contracted with the University of Colorado Medical Center to conduct an evaluation of the Utah experiment as it existed over the period from 1973 to 1975. The project was shifted to the Center for Health Services Research at the Medical Center (later termed the Health Sciences Center). In the context of the evaluation, the word "we" as employed in this book refers to the study team at the Center for Health Services Research—that is, the group of individuals who conducted the evaluation.

The evaluation was targeted at answering a number of questions, including the following:

— Was the UCIP cost-effective?

— Should it be considered on a more widespread basis?

— What were the attitudes of hospital staff, administrators, and community residents about patient care and the program in general?

— Did the program actually reduce the distance traveled by rural residents in need of long-term care?

— Did utilization of the swing-bed program differ for Medicare, Medicaid, and private-pay patients?

— What was the incremental cost of providing long-term care in hospital swing-beds?

— Did the reimbursement provided under the program actually cover the incremental cost of long-term care?

— Were acute care costs and utilization influenced by the provision of long-term care?

— How did nurses and physicians react to the program?

— Although a quality-of-care study was not formally part of this first evaluation, what inferences could be drawn regarding the quality of long-term care provided in swing-bed hospitals? Specifically, should the regulatory standards that were waived be reinstated?

The study, conducted between 1974 and 1979, involved primary data collected on-site at swing-bed hospitals, secondary data obtained from a number of sources, a variety of descriptive and multivariate statistical techniques, and interviews of providers and administrative personnel. It examined the organization, financing, and utilization of the experimental swing-bed program, and assessed the institutional capacity of rural hospitals to provide long-term care. Details, statistics, and data on the findings of the Utah swing-bed experiment can be found in the report series by Shaughnessy, Jones, et al. (1978a, 1978b). The more salient findings and implications are summarized in the rest of this chapter.

Receptivity to the Program and Related Issues and Problems

By June 30, 1973, a total of 16 hospitals had joined the experiment. During the first quarter of 1974, 9 additional hospitals, several of which had provided long-term care in hospital-based SNFs prior to the experiment, were admitted to the program. Thus, by April 1974, 25 hospitals, some of which had Medicare-certified, distinct-part SNFs, constituted the Utah experimental group of hospitals. Nineteen of these hospitals were still providing swing-bed care in 1990. The average size of the UCIP hospitals in 1974 was 37 beds, with a range from 10 to 93 beds. During 1972, the year prior to the inception of UCIP, the average UCIP hospital had 37 beds and an occupancy rate of approximately 47 percent.

Overall, we found that hospital administrators and staff reacted favorably to the UCIP experiment. Over two-thirds of the administrators felt it should be continued in rural Utah. The most frequently cited reason for the positive response by administration and staff was the benefit of the program to rural communities, providing a means to satisfy the needs of long-term care patients residing in such communities. Other frequently mentioned reasons for administrators' support of the UCIP approach were increased occupancy and increased revenues (in fact, however, revenue increases were not substantial). Some administrators felt that long-term care patients required more attention than acute care patients, although this contention was not supported by a nursing time observation study conducted as part of the evaluation.

While many physicians did not realize the swing-bed program was an experimental program in rural Utah, most viewed the swing-bed approach positively. They not only reinforced the positive attitude toward the program on the part of hospital administrators, but they also said they were able to visit long-term care patients more often in the hospital than in a nursing home because they were already at the hospital to visit acute care patients.

Whatever physician opposition existed appeared to be based on general resistance to federal and state intervention in health care. In fact, during one site visit, a physician appeared on horseback at the hospital to greet the "outside" visitors who wanted to observe the program firsthand. Astride his steed, western hat atop his head, and stethoscope slung about his neck, he unmistakenly conveyed the message that his territory was being violated by these prim and unwelcome outsiders. His comments reinforced his visual message, but also supported the new approach to long-term care for his patients. Overall, physicians appeared to become progressively more positive about the swing-bed approach over time, as the general awareness level increased about the utility of the program for patient care.

Even more so than administrators and physicians, nursing staff were strongly supportive of the swing-bed approach, citing its value to the community—and especially patients—as the primary reason for their positive attitude about the program. Some nurses, however, expressed concern that their hospital might become more of a nursing home than a hospital.

Patients and family members of patients who received long-term care under UCIP were generally satisfied with the care provided. Hospital staff, however, found that, particularly when the program was new, some patients and families had difficulty understanding that long-term care was not as intense as acute care, and they complained that they were being neglected. The staff became accustomed to explaining the implications of transferring from acute to long-term care, thus minimizing this problem.

Placement in a nursing home is often a traumatic experience for an elderly person. The idea of continuing to stay in the hospital setting after discharge from acute care turned out to be far more palatable to many patients and patient families who felt that there was a strong likelihood that the patient would eventually return home. The positive psychological impact of remaining in an acute care hospital, from which most individuals eventually return to an independent living setting, was therefore an advantage. Family members were more optimistic about the patient's future and likelihood for rehabilitation and restoration. As a result, the program was well received at the community level as word spread about the opportunity for a family member to receive long-term care services in the hospital after discharge from acute care. Despite the presence of swing beds, however, there appeared to be little impact on community nursing home occupancy rates, although this was not formally assessed as part of the evaluation of the Utah demonstration.

An issue that was to persist throughout the program was the administrators' belief that reimbursement was inadequate. More than 40 percent of the administrators felt that reimbursement provided under the experiment did not cover long-term care costs. This reaction was not surprising because it was not—and is not—traditional for administrators to think in terms of incremental cost. On the basis of administrator complaints alone, it was not clear whether reimbursement was a problem because it was truly inadequate or because it was perceived to be inadequate. The evaluation of the adequacy of reimbursement is discussed shortly.

Many administrators also reported that paperwork was excessive in the early stages of the experiment, a complaint that was due in large part to the billing requirements of Medicaid. In response to this concern, the Division of Health staff were successful in reducing the number of forms required by Medicaid, and by the end of the demonstration, complaints about paperwork appeared to approximate the level normally encountered with Medicare and Medicaid procedures.

Swing-Bed Use and Communities' Retention of Long-Term Care Patients

We also examined how swing beds were used. The analysis revealed a shift by Medicare patients from urban nursing homes to swing-bed hospitals. In 1971, of the residents of rural Utah communities who were receiving Medicare skilled nursing care in nursing homes, 64 percent were admitted to urban Medicare SNFs. Although the number of SNF admissions for residents of rural Utah increased overall, the actual number of such admissions to urban SNFs decreased substantially (by over 50 percent) with the introduction of swing beds. Some of this decrease was due to a decline in the number of Medicare-certified skilled nursing beds in urban Utah during these years. However, the decrease was primarily due to the presence of swing-beds in rural communities. By 1975, almost 70 percent of all Medicare SNF admissions for rural residents were admissions to swing-bed hospitals in rural communities.

The Utah swing-bed experiment did not have any discernible effect on acute care utilization measured in terms of acute care occupancy, length of stay, and admissions. On average, acute care occupancy rates decreased slightly for the experimental hospitals (i.e., on a before and after basis), while total hospital occupancy that included both acute care and long-term care days increased moderately. The increases in total hospital occupancy attributable to the use of hospital swing beds by long-term care patients ranged between 0 and 16 percent.

By 1975, the proportions of swing-bed days covered by different payers had stabilized. Approximately one-half of all swing-bed days were paid on an out-of-pocket basis. The remaining days were covered by Medicare and Medicaid, with Medicare covering roughly 20 percent and Medicaid covering roughly 30 percent of long-term care days in swing-bed hospitals. Since the Utah experimental program was administered by an agency closely affiliated with the Medicaid program in Utah, the question of whether Medicaid participation might be atypical in this experiment was perforce raised.

All UCIP Medicare patients and almost all UCIP Medicaid patients were classified at the skilled nursing level. Information on the level of nursing care required for private-pay patients was not available. There was reason to believe that a larger portion of Medicaid patients should have been classified either as intermediate or personal care patients, because their average length of stay was 270 days. This was greater than either the Utah or the U.S. Medicaid SNF lengths of stay for 1973 through 1975, which were 232 and 186 days, respectively. On the other hand, Medicaid intermediate care length of stay throughout Utah averaged 259 days during this period, while the Medicaid intermediate care length of stay for the entire country was 230 days. It appeared that the reason for the differences between Utah and U.S. lengths of stay for Medicaid nursing home patients rested with case-mix differences (i.e., differences in terms of patient problems and associated care needs). These differences were probably due to fewer nursing home beds per elderly in Utah, resulting in a more intense chronic care case mix, which in turn produced longer average stays for such patients. Nonetheless, the results on length of stay were surprising to some who expected shorter lengths of stay in swing beds owing to the overall acute care orientation of the hospital environment. The expectation that swing-bed providers in Utah would focus predominantly on near-acute care was not supported. In fact it was refuted by the length-of-stay findings.

Thus, there was at least an indication that the state was behaving somewhat generously toward swing-bed hospitals. As was the case with nursing homes, swing-bed hospitals were paid more for skilled patients than for intermediate or personal care patients. In any event, this finding raised the question of how typical the Utah experience would be for the sake of a decision on national swing-bed policy, which might be largely concerned with near-acute care. Since the evaluation was not designed to precisely address case-mix differences between nursing home patients and swing-bed patients, the demonstration and evaluation program did not yield sufficiently precise information for policy purposes in this area.

The Incremental Cost of Swing-Bed Care

Payment rates for swing-bed care were based on per day rates established by the Utah Medicaid program: $20, $15, and $11 for skilled, intermediate, and personal care, respectively, in 1975. Hospitals billed patients directly for swing-bed long-term care days not covered by Medicare or Medicaid. These rates pertained to routine services, which typically include the provision of the patient's room and board as well as standard services usually administered in the patient's room. Medicaid paid for ancillary services, such as radiology, laboratory, therapy, and certain operating room services, on the basis of charges billed by the hospital (although it was a less generous payer for ancillary services than Medicare). Private-pay patients also paid for ancillary services on a billed charges basis. Medicare reimbursement was similar to Medicaid reimbursement, except it entailed an incentive payment based on a calculated reduction in Medicare acute care reimbursement resulting from a savings to the Medicare program. The reimbursement approach is described in more detail in Chapter 6 and in the report by Shaughnessy, Jones, et al. (1978b).

A methodology for estimating incremental cost was developed as part of the evaluation protocol (Shaughnessy, Jones, et al. 1978a, 1978b). This approach was premised on the assumption that swing-bed reimbursement should cover the add-on, or incremental, cost of providing long-term care to patients in an acute care hospital that was already staffed and equipped to provide general hospital care. It was determined that the incremental cost of providing long-term care in swing-bed hospitals, including both routine and ancillary costs, was slightly less than $10 per day in 1975.

Hospital administrators and financial officers were not then and are not now enthusiastic about reimbursement based on incremental cost. Although the cost and reimbursement figures are considerably higher today due to inflation, hospital management and fiscal officers think in terms of full cost, not incremental cost. They argue that someone has to pay the piper—if everything is reimbursed on the basis of incremental cost, health care providers will be driven to bankruptcy. Although this is a valid point, at this stage very few health care programs are deliberately designed to provide services purely on an incremental basis, with reimbursement premised on this assumption.

Although the swing-bed program increased hospitals' revenues, it was apparent in Utah that it was not going to be a financial panacea. Most administrators liked the program because it was of genuine benefit for residents of their communities. By 1975, the swing-bed program was accounting for approximately 4 percent of total revenues. The question logically arose as to how typical this result might be, adding further support to experimenting with swing beds in other geographic areas.

Hospital Capacity to Provide Long-Term Care

As mentioned, a key feature of the Utah swing-bed demonstration involved waiving, for participating hospitals, certain Medicare regulations for skilled nursing facilities. Most notably, regulatory requirements regarding rehabilitative nursing, rehabilitation services, dental services, patient activity space, and social services were waived. On average, between 90 and 100 percent of skilled nursing facilities (i.e., Medicare-certified nursing homes) in Utah satisfied each of these five requirements. However, the experimental swing-bed hospitals complied with these requirements to a considerably lesser extent: rehabilitative nursing, 75 percent compliance; rehabilitation services, 52 percent; dental services, 52 percent; patient activity space, 37 percent; and social services, 28 percent.

The findings raised the question of whether the quality of long-term care might be lower in swing-bed hospitals relative to nursing homes, even though the presence of a variety of laboratory, diagnostic, and therapeutic services could theoretically enhance skilled nursing care in swing-bed hospitals. Again, since the evaluation was not designed to rigorously assess quality of care, the results on noncompliance further pointed to the value of another demonstration, possibly at another geographic site, to investigate this issue.

Our initial research showed no differences in diagnoses between swing-bed patients and skilled nursing patients from other Medicare-certified long-term care facilities in Utah. However, these results were qualified because medical diagnoses were used exclusively, whereas long-term care patients should also be examined in terms of functional capabilities, mental/cognitive problems, social needs, various types of chronic care problems, and emotional needs. Research on the most important attributes for analyzing long-term care case mix had not progressed very far at this point.

A nursing time study was undertaken to ascertain potential differences between acute care and long-term care patients in swing-bed hospitals. The study entailed observing nursing time spent with acute care patients and with long-term care patients in swing beds. Overall, it was found that nurses spent an average of approximately 180 minutes per day with swing-bed patients, only about 3 minutes per day more than total time spent in skilled nursing facilities throughout the United States in the mid-1970s (Shaughnessy, Jones, et al. 1978a, 1978b). Nevertheless, it was considerably less than the 310 minutes of nursing time per day spent with acute care patients in the same swing-bed hospitals. It was apparent that acute care patients received considerably more attention from nurses than did long-term care patients in swing beds. However, nursing care provided in swing-bed hospitals was characterized by greater proportions of registered nurse (RN) and licensed practical nurse (LPN) care than was the case in nursing homes, where a much higher proportion of nursing time was provided by nurses aides.

Thus, the swing-bed program was now underway thanks to the diligence of a few individuals who could see the value of a flexible approach to providing long-term care in rural areas. After several years, the program was successfully retaining elderly patients in their home communities, and rural hospitals were learning how to provide long-term care. The evaluation of the program confirmed several of the expected benefits of the swing-bed approach, but also raised further questions about the quality of long-term care, about lengths of stay of Utah swing-bed patients that implied a more chronic care than near-acute care orientation, and, overall, about generalizing from the Utah experience.

CHAPTER 2 SUMMARY

Bruce Walter first proposed the swing-bed approach as a solution to the problems of unmet demand for long-term care and oversupply of hospital beds in rural Utah in the autumn of 1969. Over the next three years, despite serious challenges to his proposal, he held steadfastly to the tenet that the approach would prove useful. The idea of providing both long-term care and acute care in hospital beds, while certainly not new when taken in a historical context, was novel in the Medicare-Medicaid era. Providing nursing home care in empty hospital beds was appealing because it might not only solve the dilemma of how to make use of such beds in rural communities, but it might even prove cost-effective if a reimbursement approach based on incremental cost was found to be acceptable.

Despite the intuitive appeal of swing beds, Medicare officials were understandably concerned that they could keep rural hospitals open unnecessarily. Further, was not the Medicare extended care facility (ECF) sufficient? If hospitals were to convert acute care beds to ECF beds in rural communities, this might solve our problems. On the other hand, proponents of the swing-bed approach argued that converting acute care beds to hospital-based ECFs, and later hospital-based skilled nursing facilities (SNFs), would reduce flexibility of bed use for small rural hospitals. In addition, converting acute care beds would actually cost Medicare and Medicaid more in the long run, assuming incremental cost reimbursement would be adequate for swing-bed care. Hospital administrators were leery of the program. In rural areas, administrators were resistant to federal intervention, and most knew little about institutional long-term care. The nursing home industry voiced concerns that the swing-bed approach would take away their patients. Officials associated with the health planning movement echoed some of the same concerns that Medicare staff voiced, particularly that this approach might contribute to retaining unnecessary hospital beds in rural communities. A general concern was voiced that hospitals might not be able to provide long-term care as well as nursing homes. This would exacerbate the already strong concerns about the quality of institutional long-term care in the United States.

Bruce Walter persevered. Medicare officials agreed that his points had merit. The Utah Cost Improvement Project (UCIP) was implemented as an experimental program to demonstrate the potential viability of the swing-bed approach in rural Utah. By 1974, 25 hospitals were enlisted in the demonstration program. Hospital beds were used to provide not only acute care, but also skilled and intermediate care with payment from Medicare and Medicaid, as well as private pay. The two main features of the experimental program involved (1) waivers of certain regulatory conditions typically necessary for nursing homes to be certified as Medicare and Medicaid providers, and (2) a reimbursement approach based on incremental cost.

Despite various start-up problems, the demonstration program proved successful from the perspective of showing that the swing-bed approach was feasible and warranted analysis on a more widespread basis. Although some expected Utah swing-bed hospitals to focus on near-acute care patients, a mix of chronic care and near-acute care patients characterized the swing-bed program. In fact, it turned out that more chronic care was provided than near-acute care.

The Bureau of Health Insurance in the Social Security Administration (later the Health Care Financing Administration) sponsored the demonstration and its evaluation, which was conducted by our research center at the University of Colorado. The evaluation study found that the approach was not only acceptable, but it proved popular with long-term care patients who received care in hospital swing beds, the families of such patients, hospital administrators, physicians, and nurses. A considerably higher proportion of patients were now receiving long-term care in their home communities throughout rural Utah. Physicians liked the program because they could visit their patients more frequently. Administrators and nurses felt that community long-term care needs were now considerably better satisfied than in the past. Patients and patient families liked the idea of being cared for in a hospital rather than a nursing home. They felt better about the more therapeutic environment of the hospital. The shorter distances that were required for family and friends to travel led to a stronger support system for long-term care patients in swing beds.

Nonetheless, the UCIP swing-bed program also raised certain questions. The average stay for Medicaid patients was 270 days, far from what would be expected if the program were focusing on near-acute care patients. Was this typical or was it because of the strong affiliation with, and support of, the swing-bed approach by the state Medicaid program? If the program were implemented elsewhere, would we see the same tendency to provide chronic care to long-stay patients, or would it result in higher numbers of near-acute care patients? While reimbursement based on incremental cost was found to be adequate by the evaluation study, would it prove acceptable in other communities? Since a formal study of the quality of long-term care provided in swing beds was not undertaken, concerns about quality persisted. Such concerns were important to address frequently, since the waived Medicare requirements for nursing homes were generally not satisfied by swing-bed hospitals. In all, the approach clearly helped satisfy a strong community need in rural areas in Utah. It appeared to do so at minimal cost, but our ability to generalize from the program was limited. As a result, the Health Care Financing Administration began to consider health policy research that might shed further light on whether and how to implement a national program.

CHAPTER 3

The Second Stage of Experimentation in Iowa, South Dakota, and Texas

THE NEXT ROUND OF SWING-BED DEMONSTRATIONS

Rationale

The Utah experience had confirmed several of the basic tenets of the swing-bed idea originally espoused by Bruce Walter. The unmet need for institutional long-term care in rural communities could be satisfied, at least in part, by using hospital beds to provide long-term care. Further, the use of surplus staff capacity in underoccupied rural hospitals seemed to render this a reasonably efficient approach in terms of resource use. Although an acclimation period was necessary, hospital staff, including physicians and nurses, accepted the approach and considered it beneficial for both patients and rural hospitals. The nursing home industry in Utah seemed to accept the swing-bed program. The expected benefits of providing long-term care in the patient's home community rather than more distant locations did occur; patients and patients' families preferred swing-bed hospitals to more distant nursing homes outside the patients' home community. The modest increases in revenues that accrued to hospitals, although not substantial, helped somewhat in diversifying and strengthening the revenue base of small rural hospitals.

Nonetheless, if the swing-bed approach were to be considered nationally, a number of policy-relevant issues still had to be addressed more specifically. It was essential to develop an appropriate mechanism for financing long-term care provided in hospital swing beds. Was the Utah reimbursement methodology acceptable in this regard? The method of paying for such care, the manner in which it would mesh with current reimbursement policy, and the financial incentives it presented for hospital providers of long-term care were likely to be strong determinants of the success of a more widespread swing-bed program.

The appropriateness of swing-bed care had to be considered in view of the unmet and still growing demand for long-term care services in many communities. Some signs were beginning to appear suggesting that the demand for near-acute care would increase over the next decade. If so, would swing-bed hospitals be a reasonable place to provide such care for residents of rural communities, or should new Medicare SNF beds be built in these communities? The lengths of stay for swing-bed patients in the Utah experiment were substantially greater than would be anticipated if the program were focusing on near-acute care. Would the Utah case-mix experience be replicated in other locations or, owing to the perhaps stronger unmet demand for chronic care in rural Utah, would we see more near-acute care provided by rural swing-bed hospitals in other states?

The swing-bed approach obviously challenged the adaptability and flexibility of our health care regulatory system. Nationally, if such a program were to be implemented, we would have to deal with issues related to health care capital expenditures regulation, certificate of need at the state level that was implemented as part of the health planning movement to restrict the supply of providers, nursing home licensure for hospitals, professional licensure for hospital administrators (since nursing home administrators must be licensed), adapting hospital reimbursement policy to incorporate swing-bed reimbursement, and the manner in which to apportion swing beds between acute and long-term care for planning and regulatory purposes. These challenges presented to the regulatory system by the swing-bed approach necessitated further scrutiny on an experimental basis in other locations.

Under the assumption that it would be possible to take advantage of existing hospital capacity to provide long-term care, the Utah experience indicated that it would be reasonable to expect that the unit cost (cost per day) of such care would be less than the unit cost of providing care in newly constructed nursing homes. However, it could also be assumed that total health care costs might increase at least slightly, since an unmet demand for long-term care appeared to exist in many rural areas. If this demand were to be met, total health care costs could likely rise even though the swing-bed program might be the most cost-effective means to meet the demand. While additional demonstrations in other states would not address this question directly, it could be an issue that might influence the viability of a national swing-bed program.

Even in the mid-1970s, the increasing trend toward quality assurance and utilization review in long-term care would raise more questions about swing beds. The results of the Utah evaluation at least suggested there was reason to be concerned that rural hospitals, many of which tended to be inexperienced in addressing the broad spectrum of behavioral, social, emotional, and functional needs of long-term care patients, were not as qualified as certified nursing homes to provide such care. Consequently, developing quality assessment, quality assurance, and utilization review programs for long-term care provided in swing beds warranted consideration.

Finally, if a swing-bed program were to be implemented nationally, a critical issue would be the specification of which hospitals would be eligible. Decisions would have to be made on whether eligibility criteria should be specified in terms of hospital occupancy rate, number of beds, geographic location (e.g., rural versus urban), and availability of certified nursing home beds in the community.

The Second Success: A New Demonstration Program

In 1975, the Social Security Administration issued a request for proposals for hospitals to participate in new swing-bed demonstrations that would further test the swing-bed approach under experimentation in Utah. Pursuant to this competitive solicitation, SSA awarded contracts to administer swing-bed demonstrations to the Texas Hospital Association and Blue Cross of Western Iowa and South Dakota (the Medicare fiscal intermediary for western Iowa and South Dakota). Owing to the reimbursement methodology, which was similar to but not the same as the Utah methodology, these demonstrations were termed the reducing acute care costs (RACC) experiments. With the award of the RACC demonstrations, SSA therefore achieved a diversity among administering organizations for the ongoing demonstrations: the state government in Utah, a fiscal intermediary in western Iowa and South Dakota, and a provider association in Texas.

In late 1975, Blue Cross of Iowa submitted an unsolicited proposal to SSA outlining an experiment similar to the RACC experiments, but with a unique reimbursement procedure. SSA awarded a contract to Blue Cross of Iowa, the Medicare fiscal intermediary for central Iowa, to administer the Iowa Swing-Bed Program (ISBP) in early 1977. Under all three experiments (UCIP, RACC, and ISBP), participating hospitals were reimbursed for long-term care using a per day payment for routine skilled nursing care that varied across the demonstrations but was constant within each. Reimbursement for ancillary long-term care was handled in accord with the normal Medicare procedure for acute care. For the UCIP and RACC demonstrations, the reimbursement approach also involved an incentive payment, which tended to encourage hospital participation in the swing-bed program. The central Iowa project differed from the first two, however, in that no incentive was included in its reimbursement formula.

As in Utah, Medicaid and private-pay patients also received long-term care in many of the participating hospitals in the RACC and ISBP experiments, although Medicaid's participation did not begin until well after the experimental programs had been implemented. Medicaid reimbursement consisted of a per day payment for skilled care in Texas and separate per day payments for skilled and intermediate care in South Dakota. Unlike Medicare, Medicaid reimbursement did not include an incentive payment in Texas and South Dakota. Ancillary reimbursement was handled in accord with standard Medicaid procedures in each state. In Iowa, Medicaid participated only to the extent of paying coinsurance for dual Medicare/Medicaid beneficiaries. As in Utah, private-pay patients were generally charged at the per diem rates used by Medicare and Medicaid and were billed for ancillary services on a fee-for-service basis.

In the final Medicare reimbursement settlement, hospital long-term routine care revenues from swing-bed care were subtracted or carved out from total routine care costs. This reduced the total Medicare allowable routine cost, resulting in the experimental name "Reducing Acute Care Costs." The RACC incentive payment to participating hospitals consisted of 50 percent of this savings, or reduction, in Medicare allowable acute care costs attributable to the provision of long-term care. The reimbursement incentive in the original swing-bed experiment in Utah was similar to, but not precisely the same as, that employed in the RACC experiments. The RACC and ISBP demonstrations involved waiving the same SNF conditions of participation waived under the Utah demonstration. The evaluation study of the Utah swing-bed program, however, had raised some questions as to the appropriateness of such waivers. The evaluation study of the new demonstrations would address this issue more directly.

Implementing the Programs

Implementation of the RACC experiment was originally scheduled to begin in January 1976. However, the first long-term care patients were not admitted to participating hospitals in either Texas or western Iowa until July 1976, and in South Dakota until August 1976. The six- to seven-month delay was due to administrative impediments in obtaining signed agreements of participation from all parties involved, complications in obtaining final approvals for the waivers of SNF conditions of participation and cost reimbursement principles, and delays in completing initial educational and training programs required for participating hospitals.

In addition, a legal controversy arose in South Dakota regarding whether that state's certificate-of-need law required participating hospitals to obtain a certificate of need prior to providing long-term care. The director of the South Dakota Comprehensive Health Planning Program (CHPP) initially indicated in a December 1975 letter to Blue Cross of Western Iowa and South Dakota that a certificate of need would not be required since long-term care was a lower level of care than acute care. The South Dakota Nursing Home Association, however, challenged the nonapplicability of certificate of need, threatening a court injunction to block implementation of the experiment. The director of CHPP, under pressure from the Nursing Home Association, reconsidered his earlier decision, and in April 1976 requested a legal opinion from the South Dakota attorney general. In July 1976, the attorney general stated that "the possible applicability of the certificate-of-need law to this situation is at best doubtful." He concluded that since there was to be no construction or modification of an existing building in any hospital as part of the swing-bed experiment, the certificate-of-need law did not apply.

SSA also required that the administering agencies obtain exemptions from nursing home licensure requirements in the participating states. For all three states, the nursing home licensure requirement was waived because acute care hospital licensure was considered to cover the less medically intense levels of care provided under the experiments.

Negotiations on establishing per diem rates for reimbursing swing-bed hospitals varied by project, although in none of the experiments did the Medicare per diem rates eventually approved by SSA exceed the Medicaid SNF rates in the project states. In Texas, SSA approved the statewide average Medicaid SNF reimbursement rate for Medicare reimbursement. After considerable discussion and negotiation, the hospitals participating in the swing-bed project in South Dakota and western Iowa were reimbursed by Medicare at a rate equal to the statewide average Medicaid SNF cost, which was not the same as the average Medicaid reimbursement rate. In central Iowa, the Medicare per diem was set at the average cost per patient day of providing skilled care in Medicare- and Medicaid-certified skilled nursing facilities.

In both of the new demonstrations, an educational program was implemented for participating hospital staff prior to admitting long-term care patients. Although the design and implementation of these programs was project specific, they shared the common focus of providing training for the hospital administrative and patient care staff members involved in the provision of long-term care. They were also intended to acquaint the general public with the swing-bed program (although this was done to varying degrees and with considerable variation in effectiveness). In meetings with hospital and administrative staff, emphasis was placed on education about financial matters, changes in Medicare cost reports, billing procedures, and the skilled nursing services that would be reimbursed under the experiments. The perceived importance of physician approval of the programs prompted emphasis on explaining the advantages of the swing-bed approach to physicians, emphasizing the role physicians would play in the success of the experiment. Training sessions in providing long-term care were conducted for nursing personnel at each of the participating hospitals. Such sessions dealt with the philosophy and practice of skilled nursing care and related topics. Public meetings were held in several communities served by the swing-bed hospitals to explain the benefits of the experiments to both hospital staff and residents of the community.

The combined RACC and ISBP demonstrations more than tripled the size of the original Utah program. In all, 83 new hospitals would participate: 39 from Texas, 22 from western Iowa and South Dakota, and 22 from central Iowa. The average numbers of beds in the participating hospitals prior to the implementation of the swing-bed demonstrations were 38 for Texas hospitals, 37 for western Iowa and South Dakota hospitals, and 62 for central Iowa hospitals. Occupancy rates averaged 44 percent for Texas hospitals, 42 percent for western Iowa and South Dakota hospitals, and 50 percent for central Iowa hospitals. In general, the hospitals participating in the swing-bed experiment tended to be smaller and characterized by lower occupancy rates than the rural hospitals in their respective states that were not participating in the swing-bed demonstrations.

RESULTS FROM THE SECOND ROUND OF DEMONSTRATIONS

The Evaluation Study

In autumn 1976, after a competitive solicitation, SSA awarded a contract to the Center for Health Services Research at the University of Colorado Health Sciences Center to evaluate the RACC and ISBP experiments.

The evaluation was to provide information on the effectiveness of the swing-bed programs in Texas, Iowa, and South Dakota, with a view toward facilitating decisions on more widespread implementation of swing-bed care. The fact that our research center was also evaluating the Utah demonstration would assist in integrating the policy implications from the two studies. The RACC and ISBP evaluation was divided into five components: organization, utilization, quality, finance, and policy.

The purpose of the organizational component was to determine whether and how a national swing-bed program should be implemented from the perspective of acceptance by hospital staff and nursing home administrators. The relationship between staff acceptance of the swing-bed approach and selected hospital and project characteristics was analyzed. Benefits of, and problems with, providing long-term care in acute care hospitals were examined, and suggestions made by both swing-bed hospital and nursing home administrators for implementation of a national swing-bed program were considered.

The utilization component of the evaluation was designed to describe the acute and long-term care utilization patterns associated with the experimental swing-bed programs. It entailed assessing the influence of the availability of swing-bed care on acute care utilization in swing-bed hospitals, and on nursing home utilization by residents of swing-bed communities. The utilization component included an analysis of case-mix differences between swing-bed and comparison nursing home patients. This component was intended to provide more specific information on the mix of near-acute care and chronic care needs of patients who used swing beds in the new experimental communities. It also included a methodology for predicting utilization patterns in the event a national swing-bed program might be implemented.

The quality of care component was intended to assess the quality of long-term care provided by the experimental swing-bed hospitals relative to that provided by Medicare- and Medicaid-certified SNFs. Site visits were made to 36 swing-bed hospitals and 15 comparison nursing homes in rural communities in Texas, Iowa, and South Dakota to collect primary data on the quality of care provided. The 15 comparison nursing homes were deliberately selected under the assumption that they provided at least average, if not above average, quality of care in comparison to other rural nursing homes. The evaluation focused on services provided to long-term care patients, not changes in patient status over time; patient outcomes were analyzed subsequently in the study of the national program in the 1980s.

The primary objective of the financial component of the evaluation was to assess the cost, both full and incremental, of providing long-term care in swing-bed hospitals. We emphasized estimating incremental cost in the evaluation for several reasons. First, the experimental approach to reimbursement was partially premised on covering incremental cost. Second, the incremental cost of long-term care in swing-bed hospitals is not only less (by definition) than full cost (an important issue for payers), but to estimate it accurately would be in keeping with the objective of taking advantage of the acute care base of the hospital to provide long-term care. Third and perhaps most important, if this new program were to be cost-effective, it would have to be competitive with nursing home care from a cost and reimbursement perspective. Finally, it was likely that reimbursement policy for any type of national program would be structured to cover incremental cost as the most acceptable, and therefore politically expedient, approach to reimbursement. The impact of the swing-bed program on the financial position of participating hospitals was also assessed, and reimbursement procedures and problems were monitored as part of this component.

The intent of the policy component of the evaluation study was to direct the analytic procedures and empirical findings of the overall evaluation toward policy-relevant conclusions by integrating the findings and implications of the four separate components described above. Topics covered in the above components—such as cost effectiveness, reimbursement policy, regulatory adaption, interpretation of utilization and cost projections in the context of a national program, and various state-level considerations—all pertained to the policy component. Hence, this component was designed to synthesize the overall study implications in terms of regulatory, reimbursement, and other health care issues, thereby providing a summary of the conclusions from a policy perspective.

A number of primary and secondary data sources were employed in the evaluation study of the RACC and ISBP swing-bed demonstrations. Further information on the data sources, data collection methods, statistical procedures, and empirical results are given in the report series resulting from the evaluation study (Shaughnessy, Tynan, et al. 1980a, 1980b). These reports document in detail the empirical findings summarized in the present chapter.

Description of and Reaction to the Program

Over 90 percent of the hospital administrators in the experimental program joined the swing-bed project to increase hospital occupancy, satisfy a need for long-term care in their communities, and use hospital space more efficiently. About two-thirds of the administrators indicated they joined in order to increase revenues. Nonetheless, it was apparent that hospitals were responding to community needs first and foremost, not solely to financial incentives or disincentives. This proved to be an important characteristic of the swing-bed approach from a policy perspective (Vladeck 1987a).

Acceptance of the swing-bed experience was relatively high for the four different types of hospital staffs surveyed. About three-fourths of hospital administrators, chiefs of staff, directors of nursing, and staff physicians wanted the experiment continued on a more permanent basis. Comparisons across the demonstration projects indicated that the central Iowa project had the highest level of acceptance among hospital staff, closely followed by the western Iowa and South Dakota project. The differences in hospital staff acceptance were related to several factors. First, more hospital administrators from Iowa and South Dakota joined the experiment to meet a need for long-term care in their communities. Second, more hospitals in these two projects had previously provided long-term care in a distinct-part SNF. Third, hospital staff attendance at orientation was higher in these two projects. Fourth, hospitals in these two projects employed more registered nurses and fewer licensed practical nurses than Texas hospitals. Lastly, central Iowa hospitals had more services available that are often needed by long-term care patients (e.g., physical therapy, speech therapy, occupational therapy, social services, and patient activities).

Most of the nursing home administrators surveyed in the demonstration states felt that a national swing-bed program should be implemented. Nursing home administrators in central Iowa were most receptive to a national swing-bed program (74 percent); those in Texas were least receptive (42 percent). A majority of hospital and nursing home administrators felt a national program should be restricted to hospitals in rural areas without a skilled nursing facility in their service area. Hospital administrators and nursing home administrators tended to disagree on the levels of care that should be allowed under a national program. Hospital administrators generally felt that both skilled and intermediate care should be included in a national program, but only one-third of nursing home administrators favored having intermediate care as part of a national program.

Once again, the benefit of swing-bed care mentioned most frequently by hospital staff members was satisfying the need for long-term care in their communities. This was reinforced by nursing home administrators who considered it beneficial for hospitals to provide long-term care when nursing home beds were unavailable. Nonetheless, nursing home administrators expressed the concern that staffing might be insufficient in swing-bed hospitals to provide both acute and long-term care.

Problems with the swing-bed program most frequently mentioned by hospital staff were inadequate reimbursement and inadequate orientation for physicians.

Utilization Findings

Contrary to the Utah experience, not all participating hospitals admitted long-term care patients to swing beds. By 1978, long-term care was being provided by 51 of the 83 rural hospitals participating in the swing-bed experiments in Texas, Iowa, and South Dakota. The average admitting hospital in South Dakota provided 1,180 days of long-term care in hospital swing beds, western and central Iowa admitting hospitals averaged about 550 days, and admitting hospitals in Texas provided slightly less than an average of 300 long-term care days in 1978. One swing-bed admitting hospital provided only 8 days of long-term care, while another provided 3,367 days.

Medicaid paid for only 3 percent of the experimental long-term care days in 1978 in the ISBP and RACC projects, an amount considerably less than the 30 percent covered by the Utah Medicaid program. Medicare reimbursed for 37 percent, and private pay for the remaining 60 percent, of the experimental long-term care days. Payer mix was substantially different between South Dakota and Texas: Medicare paid for 23 percent of the long-term care days in South Dakota, compared with 63 percent in Texas. This was largely due to the fact that the Texas hospitals provided only skilled nursing care and South Dakota hospitals provided all three levels of long-term care, including personal care (which was not reimbursable under Medicaid or Medicare). For all hospitals combined, one-half of the swing-bed care days were SNF days; the remainder of swing-bed days were predominantly intermediate care days.

For all RACC and ISBP hospitals, the average length of stay for SNF swing-bed days in 1978 was 16 days at the skilled level, considerably less than Utah. Even the average stay for personal care patients who paid exclusively on a private-pay basis was only 172 days, approximately 100 days shorter than the average stay in the Utah demonstration.

Hospitals with lower occupancy rates were found to provide more long-term care than those with higher occupancy rates. An analysis of changes in acute care occupancy over time in swing-bed hospitals and non-swing-bed comparison hospitals indicated that acute care lengths of stay decreased to a greater extent in swing-bed hospitals. These results suggested that some substitution of long-term care for acute care took place for patients in swing-bed hospitals.

Once again, however, as is clear from the total numbers of swing-bed days discussed above, the amount of long-term care provided in the experimental swing-bed hospitals was relatively small compared with acute care. Analogously, swing-bed hospitals accounted for a very small proportion of total statewide long-term care days (provided predominantly by nursing homes) during the experimental period. In South Dakota, the state with the most swing-bed days, long-term care provided in swing-bed hospitals accounted for approximately 2 percent of the total long-term care days in 1977.

Long-term care utilization was found to increase in the participating states between 1975 and 1977. Even with swing-bed hospitals providing long-term care, however, a slight increase in the occupancy of existing nursing homes tended to take place. For example, the occupancy rate for South Dakota nursing homes increased from 95 to 97 percent over this period, despite the addition of 41 new nursing home beds and the introduction of the swing-bed program. We concluded that virtually no substitution of swing-bed care for rural nursing home care took place in project communities as a result of the experiments. The results suggested that patients were very likely (1) no longer traveling to urban locations for such care—as found in Utah, (2) spending less time in acute care—substantiated by the evaluation as discussed above, (3) receiving less physician/outpatient care than previously, an issue that would later be evaluated under the national program (home health care was not widely available as an alternative in the project communities in the late 1970s), or (4) some combination of the above.

Differences between long-term care patients in swing-bed hospitals and in nursing homes in rural communities were found for a number of problem areas used to measure long-term care case mix. In general, the differences pointed to a greater tendency for nursing homes to admit patients with chronic care problems; swing-bed hospitals had a greater predisposition to admit patients with near-acute care problems. For example, various types of sensory impairments, such as impaired vision and neurological speech disorders, were more prevalent among nursing home patients. Secondary skin conditions, incontinence, and neurological immobility were also more prevalent among nursing home patients. Certain types of psychosocial problems tended to characterize nursing home patients more than swing-bed patients.

Conversely, swing-bed patients were characterized by greater independence in activities of daily living (i.e., bathing, dressing, and feeding) than nursing home patients, a pattern more characteristic of acute care patients than long-term care patients. More swing-bed patients had problems associated with pain, often from postsurgical or near-acute care problems, than nursing home patients. While some of the sample sizes were small, the patterns suggested that swing-bed patients also tended to be characterized by more near-acute problems such as shortness of breath/dyspnea and orthopedic immobility, which we found to be reflective of near-acute care problems in subsequent studies (Shaughnessy and Kramer 1990). Swing-bed hospitals tended to have more rehabilitative long-term care patients whose stays were relatively brief compared with traditional nursing home patients. Swing-bed patients more often demonstrated physical improvement, or psychological stability or improvement. At this stage of our research, we had not fully developed a profile of patient status indicators that discriminated effectively between near-acute and chronic care. However, in retrospect, the tracer indicators that were available in the data set from this evaluation suggested a proclivity toward near-acute care on the part of swing-bed hospitals relative to the chronic care provided in traditional nursing homes (Shaughnessy, Schlenker, and Polesovsky 1986; Shaughnessy, Schlenker, et al. 1985).

Quality of Care

Quality of care was measured primarily in terms of the adequacy of services provided to long-term care patients. It was measured at four different levels: for each service provided, for each individual patient problem (a patient could have several problems), for each patient, and, in the aggregate, for each facility (i.e., nursing home or hospital). The service- and problem-level quality scores were most important since they allowed for a more detailed assessment of quality and were based on higher frequencies (i.e., sample sizes). The methodology for measuring and analyzing quality is presented in more detail elsewhere (Shaughnessy, Tynan, et al. 1980a, 1980b; Shaughnessy, Breed, and Landes 1982; Shaughnessy, Schlenker, et al. 1989a, 1989b).

The quality of care provided in swing-bed hospitals was found to be lower than the quality of care provided in comparison nursing homes, using problem-level quality scores. The average nursing home problem quality score was 68 percent, and the average hospital score was 64 percent out of a maximum possible score of 100 percent. Problem-level quality scores varied greatly by problem type. Our quality scores were based on expert-derived standards of care, so that the (nearly impossible) score of 100 percent would denote perfect care in the opinion of experts in the long-term care field. Therefore, in examining swing-bed care relative to nursing home care, we focused not on the actual values, that is, 68 and 64 percent, but the difference between scores. For both nursing homes and swing-bed hospitals, psychosocial problems had the lowest quality scores. However, hospital quality scores were lower than nursing home quality scores by 20 percent in this problem area. Hospital problem quality scores were somewhat lower than nursing home scores for the specific problems of primary skin condition, urinary incontinence, depression and loneliness, and isolation and lack of socialization. When skilled nursing patients were analyzed separately, the differences in psychosocial problems lessened but remained significant. These results confirmed the expectation that the chronic, emotional, and social needs of long-term care patients were better satisfied in nursing homes than in short-stay acute care hospitals.

The more enhanced service regimens for chronic care patients in nursing homes were further evident through an analysis of specific service categories. For example, quality scores at the service level revealed that nursing homes provided better social-recreational and therapeutic–mental health services. Hospitals, however, provided better laboratory services. When service-level analyses were restricted to skilled nursing patients, swing-bed hospitals provided better physical and occupational therapies than nursing homes. In swing-bed hospitals, findings showed that skilled nursing patients received consistently higher-quality care than intermediate-level patients at the patient, problem, and service levels.

Physicians visited long-term care patients considerably more frequently in swing-bed hospitals than in comparison nursing homes. For swing-bed hospital patients, 86 percent were visited at least weekly by physicians, compared with 17 percent of the nursing home patients.

Written discharge plans were present considerably more frequently for comparison nursing home patients than swing-bed hospital patients. Nearly two-thirds of the medical charts reviewed for nursing home patients contained written discharge plans, compared with only about one-quarter of all such charts for swing-bed patients. This potential problem with discharge planning for swing-bed hospitals was compounded by the fact that a considerably higher proportion of swing-bed patients than nursing home patients were expected to be discharged within three months.

As in Utah, a substantial discrepancy was found between Medicare-certified skilled nursing facilities and swing-bed hospitals in terms of compliance with key Medicare/Medicaid conditions of participation, which were waived for the experimental hospitals. The greatest discrepancies between nursing homes and hospitals in this regard were in patient activities and social services, both of which were available with considerably greater frequency in nursing homes.

In all, the quality-of-care results showed that swing-bed hospitals were performing more poorly than nursing homes in providing traditional long-term care services typically required by patients with chronic care needs. The findings also suggested, however, that swing-bed hospitals might be performing better than nursing homes in providing restorative and rehabilitative services often required by near-acute patients with rehabilitation potential. This could only be verified, however, through a study of patient outcomes, not done as part of this evaluation. The findings and implications from the quality-of-care component of the evaluation would ultimately provide the basis for several quality assurance steps taken in the national swing-bed program. They also provided the focal points for an assessment of the quality of care in the evaluation study of the national program.

Cost and Reimbursement

In 1978, the incremental cost of routine care per long-term care patient day in the RACC and ISBP hospitals was found to be lower than the routine care reimbursement rate for such hospitals. Routine care reimbursement per long-term care patient day for certified nursing homes in Texas, Iowa, and South Dakota averaged from $5 to $15 per day more than the incremental cost of swing-bed care. The methodologies for estimating incremental costs are available elsewhere (Shaughnessy, Tynan, et al. 1980a, 1980b).

Except for a few hospitals, the experimental swing-bed program did not significantly strengthen the financial position of the participating hospitals. Long-term care revenues from routine care averaged about 3 percent of total patient care revenues in 1978. A cost-effectiveness analysis, based on the ratio of quality to incremental cost, was conducted to compare long-term care provided in swing-bed hospitals to certified nursing homes. Since the quality of long-term care was found to be only slightly higher in nursing homes than in experimental swing-bed hospitals, and since the incremental cost of long-term care in swing-bed hospitals was substantially lower than nursing home cost, the analysis indicated that the provision of long-term care in swing-bed hospitals was more cost-effective than providing institutional long-term care in nursing homes. An analogous assessment based on full cost rather than incremental cost, however, indicated that nursing homes were more cost-effective as providers of long-term care. However, since we subsequently recommended that reimbursement be based on incremental cost, swing-bed hospitals were judged cost-effective under the reimbursement approach that would be used nationally.

GROWING NATIONAL SUPPORT

Recommendations from the Two Evaluation Studies

The research on the Utah swing-bed demonstration had answered several questions and also raised several others. As a result of the evaluation of the RACC and ISBP demonstrations, however, reasonable answers to the questions arising from the Utah experience were now available. Swing-bed hospitals in other states tended to gravitate more toward shorter-stay long-term care patients than was the case in Utah. This suggested that participating hospitals in a national program would be likely to focus more on patients in need of near-acute care. The quality-of-care analysis suggested, although it did not definitively prove, that swing-bed hospitals might do as well as, or even slightly better than, nursing homes in providing long-term care to many types of near-acute care patients. It was also evident, however, that nursing homes were likely to provide chronic care services to traditional long-term care patients more effectively than swing-bed hospitals. One of the dilemmas we encountered in structuring our final recommendations was whether we should suggest that swing-bed care be restricted to certain kinds of patients. We concluded, however, that both market forces and the natural tendencies of acute care facilities to prefer to provide near-acute services rather than chronic care services would be sufficient without imposing additional regulations on the types of long-term care patients that swing-bed hospitals could admit.

On the basis of the case-mix differences we found in the RACC and ISBP evaluation, and the general tendency for patient stays to be considerably shorter in swing-bed hospitals than in nursing homes, we therefore conjectured (but without complete confidence) that most hospitals participating in a national swing-bed program would tend to provide shorter-term long-term care. In other words, swing-bed patients would tend to have briefer stays than typical long-term care patients; swing-bed hospitals would probably focus on rehabilitating patients who had even moderate potential to improve, very likely discharging patients after a relatively brief period either to an independent living environment or to a nursing home if rehabilitation were not possible. Our hesitancy in reaching this conclusion stemmed from the fact that at least a handful of swing-bed hospitals did provide chronic care to traditional long-term care patients for extended stays in swing beds. This seemed to be the exception rather than the rule, however, and usually occurred appropriately in those communities where a shortage of traditional nursing home beds existed.

We knew hospital administrators were far from enamored with swing-bed reimbursement based on the incremental cost of routine care. On the other hand, our analyses had shown that such reimbursement, while not generous, was adequate and in the best interest of cost-effective patient care. In terms of effectiveness, we were confident that a national swing-bed program would greatly enhance access to near-acute long-term care services for residents of rural communities. In terms of the quality of care, our assessment of the RACC and ISBP swing-bed programs had shown that nursing homes did better, especially in providing traditional long-term care services. Yet hospitals were not substantially worse (quality scores of 68 percent versus 64 percent for nursing homes versus swing-bed hospitals), and very likely some learning would occur that would further reduce this difference.

It was beyond the scope of our quality-of-care study to examine patient outcomes, especially to determine whether patients requiring near-acute care had comparable outcomes when admitted to swing beds and to nursing home beds. Quite frankly, one of our biggest regrets was that neither of our first two evaluation studies had examined this. But outcomes of care were simply not being analyzed very much in the 1970s, especially changes in patient status over time in long-term care settings—other health policy issues were considered more important.

While the swing-bed approach might have potentially worked in urban areas, no one had any experience whatsoever with urban swing-bed hospitals. Further, the health care delivery system in urban areas is considerably more complex in terms of the range of provider types and their relative proximity to individual patient residences. Generally speaking, competition among health care providers is stronger than in rural areas, and urban health care delivery systems are characterized by both greater diversity and complexity. We knew the swing-bed approach could be reasonably successful in rural areas and were unsure of its potential success in metropolitan communities. We did not feel, however, that the swing-bed program should be restricted only to smaller hospitals in rural communities. Rural hospitals responded predominantly to community needs in providing long-term care in swing beds, taking into consideration the extent to which acute care patients already occupied such beds (i.e., we found a negative association between swing-bed hospital acute care occupancy rates and total days of swing-bed care). In fact, the state of the art in measuring outcomes in the long-term care field (from a research perspective) was still very much in its infancy at that time, so it is questionable whether definitive conclusions about patient outcomes would have been attainable.

As a result, our final evaluation report from the RACC and ISBP projects contained the recommendation that a national swing-bed program be established in rural communities throughout the United States. This recommendation was premised on the following factors:

1. the unmet demand for long-term care that existed in many rural communities

2. the assumption that satisfying this demand is socially desirable and would enhance the public welfare

3. the conclusion that many rural hospitals can and will provide

such care in an adequate manner if proper quality assurance steps are taken

4. the fact that the cost of swing-bed care would not exceed the cost of comparable care provided in other settings

Our evaluation studies were not designed, however, to analyze the cost effectiveness of every possible alternative for providing long-term care in rural communities. The most realistic and available alternative at that time for rural communities, nursing home care, was examined. The recommendations were thus premised on assessing the demand for, and cost of, the two most pragmatic alternatives for long-term care in rural communities, as well as the quality of care associated with each alternative.

The recommendations were based on our best judgment of how to proceed. Available evidence from the evaluation studies was useful but not perfect: some differences existed among the experiments, the experimental hospitals were located in small midwestern communities, and our participating hospitals were smaller and had lower occupancy rates than most rural hospitals. Our recommendations either took such factors into consideration or were qualified accordingly. Pragmatically speaking, we judged it unnecessary to call for yet more demonstrations in other rural locations since the main policy issues had been addressed reasonably carefully, and it was time to implement a national program on the basis of the results.

Using largely the results of our research on the Iowa, South Dakota, and Texas demonstrations, taken in the context of the initial Utah experiment, we recommended the following:

1. Rural hospitals (of any size) throughout the country should be allowed to provide swing-bed care.

2. Participating hospitals should be eligible to receive Medicare and Medicaid reimbursement for long-term care provided in swing beds.

3. Individual states should be permitted to impose further restrictions through the certificate-of-need process (and by implication, the licensure process).

4. Medicare and Medicaid reimbursement should be structured to ensure that the incremental cost of long-term care provided in swing beds would be covered.

5. An appropriate way to cover the incremental cost of providing long-term care in swing beds would be to establish a per diem reimbursement rate using nursing home cost experience, along with an offset or a revenue carve-out method for acute care

reimbursement (but not paying an additional incentive based on the offset), thereby providing for a reasonably cost-effective approach for all payers, including private payers.

6. Medicare reimbursement for ancillary services should be handled according to standard Medicare procedures—as done in the demonstrations.

7. Medicaid reimbursement procedures should be similar to Medicare, but states should be free to structure Medicaid payment according to their own practices.

8. Hospitals should be required to satisfy some, but not all, of the Medicare/Medicaid conditions of participation that regulate SNFs.

9. In this regard, in addition to hospital certification requirements, SNF conditions of participation should be satisfied in the areas of social services, staff development, discharge planning, and patient activities (but without burdening hospitals with additional capital costs in this area).

10. Hospital-based long-term care provided in swing beds should be subject to any professional standards review organization (PSRO) requirements and Medicaid review procedures for long-term care that might be in place nationally.

11. Orientation and information dissemination would be critical to the success of a national swing-bed program, especially in terms of patient care practices and overall program management:

    a. Clearly written and prototypical guidelines for physicians and nurses on providing long-term care and the differences between long-term care and acute care should be available and disseminated.

    b. Analogously, administrative guidelines detailing reimbursement policy, forms completion, and anticipated hospital-level problems should be disseminated to hospital administrators.

Although it was not possible to precisely estimate the utilization that would occur if a swing-bed program were implemented nationally, we at least tried to give some approximate figures. The forecasting methodology used is documented in the final evaluation report (Shaughnessy et al. 1980b). Several factors made it difficult to forecast utilization:

1. Payers participated to differing degrees across the various experiments.

2. The distribution of patients within levels of long-term care varied from project to project.

3. Reimbursement procedures differed.

4. Administrative practices differed at both the hospital and state levels.

5. It was not possible to stipulate the precise eligibility and regulatory conditions that might be associated with a national program.

Nonetheless, we forecast that if the program were implemented nationally using our recommended eligibility criteria of location in a rural area and satisfaction of state certificate-of-need requirements, swing-bed utilization in rural hospitals would likely total between 750,000 and 1,971,000 long-term care days per year when the program reached its steady state—which we felt would probably be within two years following its implementation. This would represent only a 0.2 to 0.6 percent increase in institutional long-term care nationally.

Using similar forecasting procedures, we estimated that the total cost of the program in its steady state would be between $14.2 and $37.0 million in 1978 dollars. These additional costs would represent an increase of between 0.02 and 0.05 percent in total hospital expenditures nationally.

The research showed that implementation problems should be expected in several areas. The offset or carve-out method of incremental cost reimbursement recommended in the evaluation report (and used in the ISBP demonstration) was novel in the hospital setting. We cautioned that this type of reimbursement would appear inequitable from the perspective of many hospitals. Because of this, we emphasized that reimbursement policy be clearly stated, straightforward, and preferably well understood from the outset. It was apparent that hospital medical, nursing, and administrative staff would have certain difficulties adjusting to the different health care needs and service requirements of long-term care patients. Greater emphasis on rehabilitative and maintenance services associated with long-term care and the psychosocial nature of many long-term care problems would require adjustments by hospital staff. We felt that such adjustments should naturally be expected to occur over the course of time.

The demonstration and evaluation program also showed it would be reasonable to expect initial resistance to the swing-bed approach in many rural communities. Such resistance would arise from a natural aversion to federal intervention, the attitude on the part of some that an acute care hospital should not become a nursing home, and a general concern about the changing role of acute care hospitals. We advised policymakers that a national swing-bed program should be voluntary and supportive of an expanded referral network among swing-bed hospitals and nursing homes. We also recommended that should Congress decide to implement a national swing-bed program, the experimental programs in place should be continued until the implementation date of the national program.

Increased Popular Support for a National Swing-Bed Program

By the late 1970s, the swing-bed program had become popular not only in the experimental communities, but also in other selected rural areas throughout the country that had underoccupied hospitals and yet were experiencing a shortage of institutional long-term care. For example, North Dakota had already been experimenting with a private-pay swing-bed program. A number of members of Congress, especially from states with proportionately larger rural populations, had become interested in the swing-bed approach. Several bills that would create a national swing-bed program were introduced by various members of Congress in 1978 (H.R. 13817 and H.R. 5285), 1979 (H.R. 4000, H.R. 3460, H.R. 3463, S. 505, S. 507, H.R. 934, and H.R. 4480), and 1980 (S. 2468) (AHA 1979a, 1979b). The evaluation reports from the Texas, Iowa, and South Dakota demonstrations were first released in 1979 (Shaughnessy, Huggs, et al. 1979; Landes et al. 1979), complementing the reports from the Utah evaluation that were first released in early 1978 (Shaughnessy, Jones, et al. 1978a, 1978b).

By this time, HCFA staff and the administration were openly supportive of a national swing-bed approach in rural areas. Several individuals from HCFA had invested a considerable amount of time and energy in designing the swing-bed demonstrations and emphasizing that they be objectively and thoroughly evaluated. The American Hospital Association had become actively involved in supporting the swing-bed movement, monitoring and supporting various bills to implement swing-bed care nationally. Our evaluation team wrote a position paper basically discussing the pros and cons of the swing-bed approach and summarizing our recommendations for a national program. Testimony on swing-bed care was given to various congressional committees by a wide variety of individuals—by hospital staff that had participated in the provision of such care, AHA representatives, citizens supportive of the concept, HCFA officials, and our research team. The empirical evidence in support of the swing-bed approach was abundant. While the nursing home industry continued to oppose the swing-bed concept formally, its opposition was not substantial, possibly because at least a number of nursing home administrators and operators felt the program had merit for the adequate provision of long-term care in rural communities. The stage was now set with a positive predisposition toward swing-bed care on the part of Congress and the administration.

CHAPTER 3 SUMMARY

At a time when the Utah swing-bed demonstration was answering certain questions regarding the feasibility of the swing-bed approach, others were being raised that the Utah demonstration and evaluation program were not able to answer. Consequently, in 1976 and 1977 SSA implemented two new demonstration projects in Texas, Iowa, and South Dakota. The first, termed the Reducing Acute Care Costs (RACC) project, involved rural hospitals from Texas, South Dakota, and western Iowa. Hospitals from rural communities in central Iowa participated in the second, termed the Iowa Swing-Bed Project (ISBP). While these demonstrations were similar to the Utah project, there were several differences. The new demonstrations were in locations with different demographic and health care profiles (increasing the total number of hospitals participating in the swing-bed demonstration program to about 100), they were administered by different types of agencies, the approach to reimbursement was somewhat different from Utah, and they had the initial Utah experience from which to learn. In addition, our evaluation study would examine new issues that were not addressed in the original Utah evaluation.

As in Utah, the swing-bed approach in the new communities was well-received by hospital administrators, chiefs of medical staff, directors of nursing, staff physicians, nursing staff, patients, and patient families. Providers were generally pleased with the program because they felt it satisfied an unmet need for long-term care in their rural communities. A majority of nursing home administrators in the swing-bed communities in the three states felt the program should be continued and expanded to a national level. Nursing home administrators felt the program would be useful in areas where there was an inadequate supply of nursing home beds to meet community needs.

The highest utilization of swing beds for long-term care occurred in South Dakota. Even in that state, however, the average hospital provided only 1,180 days of long-term care per year in hospital swing beds. Thus, it continued to be a modest-sized program, targeted primarily at meeting the needs of community residents for long-term care that either were not being satisfied or could only be satisfied in distant nursing homes. Unlike Utah, where Medicaid covered 30 percent of long-term care patient days, only 3 percent of long-term care days in hospital swing beds were covered by Medicaid in the new demonstrations. Medicare paid for 37 percent, with the remainder of days covered by private pay. Some substitution of long-term care for acute care appeared to take place, since acute care lengths of stay decreased more in swing-bed hospitals than in comparable hospitals without swing beds.

Substantially different from Utah was the near-acute care orientation of the swing-bed hospitals in Iowa, South Dakota, and Texas. Stays for patients requiring SNF care averaged only 16 days. Even patients receiving personal care (provided only in South Dakota) had stays of but 170 days, approximately 100 days less than the average stay for all patients receiving long-term care in swing beds in Utah. A comparison of long-term care patients in community nursing homes and hospital swing beds revealed significant differences. Nursing home patients typically had more chronic care needs in the areas of sensory impairments, neurological speech disorders, incontinence, and neurological immobility. Swing-bed patients generally tended to be less dependent in functioning (i.e., more similar to acute care patients) and had more problems such as postsurgical pain, dyspnea/shortness of breath (found to be an indicator of near-acute care needs in subsequent studies), and orthopedic immobility. It was apparent that swing-bed hospitals in the new demonstration program had focused largely on near-acute care.

Quality of long-term care provided in swing-bed hospitals was compared with the quality of community nursing home care using process measures of quality, thereby assessing the adequacy of services provided to patients. Overall, the quality of long-term care provided in swing-bed hospitals was lower than the quality of long-term care provided in comparison nursing homes. The higher-quality care for nursing homes was largely attributable to better care provided to chronic care patients who require basic maintenance and supportive care in the general areas of functional, cognitive, emotional, and social needs. The results suggested, however, that various types of services required for near-acute care were better provided in swing-bed hospitals. Since swing-bed hospitals in this second round of demonstrations generally tended to provide more near-acute than chronic care, it appeared that they may have been providing adequate care to the types of patients on whom they tended to concentrate. However, considerably fewer swing-bed patient records contained written discharge plans relative to records for nursing home patients. This was of concern because swing-bed patients generally had shorter stays and higher discharge rates than nursing home patients.

Physicians continued to visit patients significantly more often in swing-bed hospitals than nursing homes. Most patients in swing-bed hospitals received at least one physician visit per week—far more than nursing home patients. The results of analyzing quality of care led us to conclude that long-term care for the types of patients typically treated in hospital swing beds was adequate and possibly even above average, but that chronic care for patients with maintenance and even palliative care needs potentially required improvement. These conclusions would form the basis for our quality assurance recommendations in the national program.

The incremental cost of swing-bed care was estimated using different methodologies. Overall, the reimbursement approach used in the demonstration was judged to yield sufficient revenues to cover the incremental cost of long-term care provided in hospital swing beds. For the most part, the swing-bed program did not substantially enhance the financial position of swing-bed hospitals. Routine care revenues from long-term care patients in hospital swing beds represented approximately 3 percent of total patient care revenues for hospitals that admitted swing-bed patients. Under the assumption that a national program might be implemented with reimbursement based on incremental cost, the swing-bed approach was found to be cost-effective. This conclusion followed from the findings that quality of care was but slightly lower in swing-bed hospitals relative to nursing homes (although quality was perhaps higher for near-acute swing-bed patients), yet incremental cost was lower than nursing home cost.

Although the swing-bed demonstration and research programs left some questions partly unanswered, both we and others felt the weight of the evidence available now called for a health policy change nationally. We made concrete recommendations on how a national swing-bed program should be structured. The recommendations dealt with rural hospital eligibility, Medicare and Medicaid participation, reimbursement, certification and regulation, certificate-of-need applicability, quality assurance, information dissemination, and guidelines for administrators and providers of care. Concurrent with, and shortly after, the release of the evaluation study reports on the various swing-bed demonstrations, governmental, provider, and popular support for the swing-bed approach gained considerable momentum.

Between 1978 and 1980, ten separate bills were introduced in Congress that contained hospital swing-bed provisions. HCFA staff and others from the administration advocated that the swing-bed approach be implemented. The HCFA recommendations generally followed from the demonstration and evaluation experience gained through the projects HCFA had funded in the 1970s. The American Hospital Association lobbied strongly in support of swing-bed enabling legislation. Our research staff wrote a position paper elucidating the recommendations that followed from our research. Congressional testimony was given by hospital staff that had participated in the swing-bed demonstrations, representatives of the American Hospital Association, private citizens, HCFA officials, and our research team. In late 1980, the Omnibus Budget Reconciliation Act would yield the fruits of the labor started by Bruce Walter a decade before.

CHAPTER 4

The National Swing-Bed Program: The First Years

ENABLING LEGISLATION AND REGULATIONS

The 1980 Law

Section 904 of the Omnibus Budget Reconciliation Act (OBRA), passed on December 5, 1980 (P.L. 96-499), contained the enabling legislation for a national swing-bed program in rural communities throughout the United States. Noteworthy in the law were the following provisions:

— Reimbursement methods for routine and ancillary services would be basically the same as those recommended in the evaluation report and used in the Iowa Swing-Bed Program.

— "The Secretary may not enter into an agreement under this section with any hospitals unless—(1) . . . the hospital is located in a rural area and has less than 50 beds, [and] (2) the hospital has been granted a certificate of need for the provision of long-term care from the State Health Planning and Development Agency . . . for the state in which the hospital is located."

— "A hospital which enters into [a swing-bed agreement] shall be required to meet those conditions applicable to skilled nursing facilities relating to discharge planning and the social services function. . . . Services furnished by such a hospital which would otherwise constitute post-hospital extended care services if furnished by a skilled nursing facility, shall be subject to the same requirements applicable to such services when furnished at a skilled nursing facility except for those requirements the

Secretary determines are inappropriate in the case of these services being furnished by a hospital under this section."

— "The Secretary may enter into an agreement under this section on a demonstration basis with any hospital which does not meet the requirement of Subsection (b)(1) [i.e., the 50-bed limit and/or location in a rural area], if the hospital otherwise meets the requirements of this section."

— "Within three years after the enactment of this Act, the Secretary . . . shall submit . . . a report evaluating the programs established by the amendments made by this section and shall include in such report an analysis of—

(1) the extent and effect of the agreements under such programs on availability and effective and economical provision of long-term care services,

(2) whether such programs should be continued,

(3) the results of any demonstration projects conducted under such programs, and

(4) whether eligibility to participate in such programs should be extended to other hospitals, regardless of bed size or geographic location, where there is a shortage of long-term care beds."

— "The amendments made by this section shall become effective on the date on which final regulations, promulgated by the Secretary to implement such amendments, are first issued; and those regulations shall be issued not later than the first day of the sixth month following the month in which this Act is enacted."

In addition, Section 903 of the same law included the following provision that pertained to the ongoing swing-bed demonstrations in Utah, Texas, Iowa, and South Dakota: "In the case of any State which has had such a demonstration project reimbursement system in continuous operation since July 1, 1977, the Secretary shall provide . . . for continuation of reimbursement to hospitals in the State under such system. . . ." This provision permitted the swing-bed demonstration hospitals to continue providing long-term care until the national program was initiated under new regulations.

The enabling legislation therefore not only established a national swing-bed program in rural areas, but it gave the secretary of Health and Human Services (HHS) the authority to expand the program to larger rural hospitals and urban hospitals on a demonstration basis. In fact, however, this demonstration authority has yet to be used by the secretary. The legislation also provided for an evaluation of the national program to determine whether it should be expanded, refined, or eliminated. As will be discussed, a national evaluation study was conducted. Its results are discussed in the next two chapters in order to describe swing-bed care as it is currently provided in the United States.

The Regulations

The regulations for the national program were delayed, not appearing until July 20, 1982. Although promulgated later than the six-month period required by Congress in Section 904, they were comprehensive and, in the opinion of many observers, exhibited a thorough knowledge of swing-bed issues. At this time, they were published in interim final form. Although comments on the regulations were solicited and received, no changes were made to the initial regulations with the exception of reimbursement amendments published on September 1, 1983.

The legislation and regulations laid the groundwork for a national swing-bed program that would be highly similar to that recommended on the basis of the research documented in the 1979 and 1980 evaluation reports. It was apparent that the experience with the demonstration programs of the 1970s had strongly shaped the national program of the 1980s. In particular, statutory and regulatory requirements, along with practices adopted as a result of such requirements, dictated that the national program would have the following characteristics (which, for comparative purposes, parallel the 11 recommended by the evaluation study, as summarized in the preceding chapter):

1. All rural hospitals with fewer than 50 beds should be allowed to provide swing-bed care, with the secretary of HHS permitting rural hospitals with greater than 50 beds to provide swing-bed care on a demonstration basis.
2. Such hospitals are eligible to receive Medicare and Medicaid reimbursement for long-term care provided in swing beds, with individual state Medicaid programs determining whether they wish to participate in the national swing-bed program.
3. Individual states are permitted to impose further restrictions through the certificate-of-need process.
4. Medicare and Medicaid reimbursement is premised on covering the incremental cost of long-term care provided in swing beds.

5. This was accomplished by establishing that the per day Medicare reimbursement rate for SNF care would be the statewide Medicaid SNF rate for the preceding year, along with a revenue offset or carve-out method for acute care reimbursement.

6. Medicare reimbursement for ancillary services would be the same as that used in the demonstration projects (basically the same as ancillary reimbursement for acute care hospitals).

7. Medicaid programs would have some flexibility in structuring their own analogous approaches to reimbursement for swing-bed care.

8. Certain SNF conditions of participation were waived for hospitals on the assumption that they were unnecessary in an acute care environment.

9. SNF conditions of participation in the following areas were required: social services and the necessary staff, patient activities (without requiring that hospitals incur unnecessary additional capital costs through construction or expansion), discharge planning, patients' rights, specialized rehabilitation services, and dental services.

10. No specific provisions on PSRO or Medicaid review procedures were contained in the initial law or regulations.

11. No specific orientation or information dissemination provisions were required or encouraged outside of the normal Medicare and Medicaid procedures.

In addition, even after the regulations were finalized, hospitals participating in the ongoing demonstration programs were allowed to continue to provide swing-bed care until the formal implementation of the national program. Although no formal guidelines or regulations on information dissemination were contained in the enabling legislation or ensuing regulations, the information dissemination approaches recommended as a result of the demonstration and evaluation studies would subsequently be provided through another source that took an interest in the national program—the Robert Wood Johnson Foundation (discussed shortly).

The federal regulations were positive in tone, connoting an understanding of the dilemmas rural hospitals would encounter in implementing a new approach to providing long-term care in hospital swing beds. As stated in the regulations (HCFA 1982, p. 31520):

> In determining which additional standard to apply, we believe that equity among providers of nursing home care requires as much consistency in

treatment as possible. For example, if certain professional services are not readily available in a particular geographic area, it seems inequitable to require that these services be provided in local freestanding and distinct part nursing homes, but not in a nearby swing-bed hospital. We have, however, kept the swing-bed requirements to a minimum, and the standards which we are including will be applied as flexibly as possible. We believe that swing-bed hospitals may have a lower daily census of long-term care patients than do nursing homes and that patients in swing-bed hospitals are less likely to become long-term care residents. We will consider these factors when surveying for compliance with the requirements.

Thus, the regulations were premised on two important attributes of swing-bed care that were evident from the demonstration period: the relatively low volume of such care provided by participating hospitals and the considerably shorter stays for swing-bed patients (relative to nursing home patients) owing to the greater prevalence of near-acute care patients in swing beds.

Although the conditions and requirements contained in legislation and regulations were highly similar to those we recommended on the basis of our research, no pretense is made that our work was the exclusive, or even dominant, force in influencing swing-bed policy. The many organizations and individuals mentioned in the preceding chapters—including providers and the provider community, HCFA staff who monitored the demonstration and evaluation programs, congressional staff and members of Congress who wrote and passed the legislation, and HCFA staff who wrote the regulations—all played major roles. Some of this work was done prior to the availability of—or at least in some cases, independently of—our research. On the other hand, it appears that the research findings both confirmed the approach as cost-effective and provided a substantive catalyst for the policy changes that ensued.

The Evaluation Study of the National Swing-Bed Program

Due to the delay in promulgating the final regulations for the program, the Office of Research and Demonstrations (ORD) at HCFA was required to wait until October 1983 to begin the congressionally requested evaluation study. This study was also competitively awarded to the Center for Health Services Research at the University of Colorado Health Sciences Center. The evaluation was designed to meet the requirements specified by Congress in Section 904 of OBRA 1980. Its specific objectives are described in more detail in the following section. HCFA twice augmented this study with additional components. One of the augmentations was designed to assess the manner in which the swing-bed program was affected by and interacted with Medicare's prospective payment system (PPS) for hospitals implemented in 1983. The second was intended to assess the effects of peer review organization (PRO) review on swing-bed hospitals relative to Medicare-certified nursing homes and home health agencies.

THE ROBERT WOOD JOHNSON FOUNDATION (RWJF) MODEL SWING-BED PROGRAM

Nature of the RWJF Model Program

The feasibility of the swing-bed approach had already been established in the late 1970s. After the enabling legislation for the early swing-bed approach was passed and regulations promulgated in the early 1980s, the major issues focused on whether and how rural hospitals could constructively implement swing beds in a new health care environment. These issues needed to be addressed given that a reimbursement system for swing-bed care was now in place, and in view of concerns about quality assurance that had been raised in the earlier demonstration programs. Further, although not yet apparent, the hospital sector in the United States was about to encounter (in PPS) the most far-reaching reimbursement and resultant patient care changes since the implementation of Medicare and Medicaid in the 1960s.

Shortly after the passage of the enabling legislation for the national swing-bed program in 1980, RWJF decided to become involved in assisting rural hospitals to implement the swing-bed approach. It established a program to develop "model swing-bed hospitals" whose initial experience would help other rural hospitals to provide swing-bed care under the new national program (Richardson and Kovner 1985, 1986, 1987). The project was intended to shape the manner in which swing-bed care would be provided in rural communities. It funded several state hospital associations and selected hospitals from these states to develop prototypical approaches to swing-bed care under the new national program.

The model program was administered for RWJF by New York University (NYU) with an advisory committee comprised of individuals representing the fields of rural health care, long-term care, swing-bed care, quality assurance, medicine, nursing, hospital administration, reimbursement policy, and research. Over the five-year duration of the RWJF program, grantee hospital associations provided a range of services to grantee hospitals and other rural hospitals interested in swing-bed care in their states. A competitive solicitation was issued by RWJF so that state hospital associations with hospitals eligible for the swing-bed program would respond with proposals for implementing model programs at the state level.

By the beginning of 1983, 5 hospital associations and 26 hospitals had been funded as part of the project. The 26 hospitals—6 each from New Mexico and Kansas, 5 each from North Dakota and Missouri, and 4 from Mississippi—had been selected and funded to serve as precursors whose experience might be of value to other rural hospitals interested in providing swing-bed care under the national program. The five state hospital associations were funded to provide both technical assistance and overall guidance to the grantee hospitals within their own states, as well as other rural nongrantee hospitals in their states. Beyond this, the state hospital associations were expected to disseminate information to other states regarding swing-bed care, dealing with the necessary approvals for reimbursement, regulatory requirements, and the like. The hospital associations in the five states were active in obtaining Medicaid participation in their states as well. Many of the initial issues regarding certificate of need, communication with fiscal intermediaries, Medicare reimbursement and certification, quality assurance, personnel management, community relations, publicity, integration with nursing homes, staff education, diversification, and provision of long-term care, were dealt with first in the model states, with information available to other hospitals and associations thereafter.

The 26 individual hospitals received grant support from RWJF to employ swing-bed coordinators (to initiate and integrate care plans and programs for swing-bed patients), establish procedures and policies for swing-bed care that might be disseminated to other hospitals, support attendance of staff at orientation workshops, acquire consulting assistance in implementing swing-bed programs, disseminate information to their communities, and in general, efficiently implement swing-bed approaches that might serve as templates for other hospitals. Staff from the grantee hospital associations and individual hospitals would eventually make presentations at workshops for nongrantee hospitals in grantee states and later in nongrantee states.

The Section for Small or Rural Hospitals of the American Hospital Association cosponsored the RWJF model program, publishing a planning guide for rural hospitals interested in swing-bed care in 1984 (Supplitt 1984). The planning guide (currently being updated by AHA) was directed toward hospitals interested in learning more about, and possibly implementing, the swing-bed approach. Many of the authors of the planning guide were on or affiliated with the RWJF/NYU advisory committee for the model program, representing a cross-section of individuals experienced in providing and administering swing-bed care; reimbursing for swing-bed care; evaluating or participating in the demonstration programs from the 1970s; and knowledgeable about rural hospitals, rural hospital issues, and long-term care. The AHA periodical, *Hospitals,* devoted several feature articles to the topic of swing-bed care shortly after the initial regulations were published (AHA 1982). Topics such as diversification opportunities, quality assurance, reimbursement, and planning for swing-bed care were covered in the special issue. An overview of swing-bed care was provided along with background information for hospitals considering the approach.

The RWJF demonstration was quite out of the ordinary. Rarely, at best, do we fund health care providers to attempt to efficiently and effectively develop an approach to implementing a new national program at a grassroots level (in specific communities). The idea behind the RWJF program was to enable selected hospitals to start providing swing-bed care reasonably quickly so that the good and bad experiences they had under the new national program might be constructively disseminated to other hospitals interested in providing swing-bed care under the very same rules and regulations (i.e., not those of an earlier demonstration program). In view of this objective, it turned out to be fortuitous that the national program started somewhat slowly.

Evaluation of the RWJF Model Project

Shortly after HCFA funded our Center for Health Services Research at the University of Colorado to evaluate the national program in late 1983, RWJF also funded our research center to evaluate their model demonstration program. With RWJF and HCFA cofunding the overall evaluation, the total national evaluation was now intended to be a balanced assessment of swing-bed care throughout the country. HCFA's primary interest was appropriately determined by the congressional mandate in the enabling legislation; RWJF's primary concern was centered on the quality of swing-bed care and, to a lesser extent, the effects of their model program on swing-bed care nationally.

The jointly funded evaluation study was designed to answer questions in six distinct areas:

1. *Participation and use.* What are the patterns of participation and use that characterize hospital involvement in the national swing-bed program, and what factors are associated with or influence such patterns? For example, what influence did the RWJF program have on the growth and nature of swing-bed participation and use?

2. *Case mix.* Does the case mix of long-term care patients who receive care in swing-bed hospitals nationally differ from the case mix of nursing home patients in the same types of communities? Would the findings from the demonstration projects regarding case-mix differences typify the new national pro-

gram? Would swing-bed hospitals throughout the country grav-itate toward providing near-acute care, or would they compete more directly with nursing homes for chronic care patients?

3. *Quality of care.* Is the quality of long-term care provided to pa-tients in hospital swing beds adequate? What are the short- and long-run outcomes of care for swing-bed patients compared with nursing home patients?

4. *Cost.* What is the cost of swing-bed care relative to nursing home care? Is the national reimbursement approach adequate to cover the cost of swing-bed care at the hospital level?

5. *PPS impacts.* How has the swing-bed program been affected by and interacted with PPS?

6. *Viability of swing-bed care.* Do the findings in the above areas indicate that the swing-bed program should be continued or expanded? What should be our short-run and long-run national policies regarding swing-bed care?

Several of the questions the national evaluation study addressed were similar to those asked during the demonstration programs. None-theless, since the demonstration programs were restrictive in terms of geographic location and types and numbers of hospitals participating, we did not know how well the demonstration and evaluation results would forecast the nature of the national program. Of particular interest was the extent to which the program would grow, the types of long-term care patients that it would serve, and the quality of care that would be provided—especially in view of the slightly enhanced care available in nursing homes relative to swing-bed hospitals in the demonstration projects.

POLICY INITIATIVES THAT INFLUENCED
THE NATIONAL SWING-BED PROGRAM

Intervening and Inhibiting Policies and Activities

Despite the positive climate for swing-bed care created by the encourag-ing tone of the federal regulations, the RWJF demonstration program, and the initial information dissemination efforts of AHA, other emerging national policies and practices would initially inhibit (and later stimulate) the growth of the national swing-bed movement. A number of significant changes in hospital reimbursement policy under Medicare were enacted under the Tax Equity and Fiscal Responsibility Act (TEFRA, P.L. 97-248) in September 1982 (Shaughnessy and Schlenker 1986). Under this law, cost limits that pertained to routine care under Section 223 of the Social Security Act were waived for small hospitals. However, such hospitals now had to comply with a new cost limit (termed the "rate-of-increase cap") that resulted in a limit on total cost per discharge for the facility. Had the previous Section 223 limits continued to be applicable to routine care alone, the swing-bed approach would have been advantageous to hospitals. However, the new limit in the form of a per discharge rate-of-increase cap under TEFRA complicated assessing the relative advantages of the swing-bed approach from a reimbursement perspective, since this pertained to total cost per discharge.

Prior to TEFRA, hospital-based and freestanding SNFs operated under separate Medicare reimbursement limits. The dual reimbursement limits were eliminated under TEFRA, reducing reimbursement for a large number of hospital-based SNFs. This further increased the degree of uncertainty associated with the incentives and disincentives of hospitals to become involved in long-term care. As a result, small rural hospitals understandably adopted a rather conservative posture due to the sweeping changes in hospital reimbursement under TEFRA. Such a posture was far from conducive to diversifying and expanding into health care programs characterized by new and different service offerings from those traditionally provided by small rural hospitals.

Less than one year after TEFRA had passed, the Social Security Amendments of March 1983 (P.L. 989-21) ushered in a new era in hospital reimbursement under PPS. This legislation radically changed hospital reimbursement and brought about a further retrenchment on the part of small rural hospitals with respect to incentives to innovate and experiment with long-term care. Hospital payment under Medicare would henceforth not be based on the cost of each *day* of care provided. Rather, it would be based on a price (related to cost) that Medicare would pay for a hospital *stay*, with payment varying according to the types of patients (diagnosis-related groups, or DRGs, were established to classify patients and determine payment). Over time, however, it became apparent that as hospital lengths of stay decreased under DRG reimbursement, the need for near-acute long-term care programs would increase. In fact, swing-bed reimbursement was based on a cost-related per diem for routine care, which would be paid upon discharge from acute care to swing-bed care. Hospitals could therefore collect their DRG payment for acute care *and* a per diem for swing-bed care thereafter. The combined PPS and swing-bed payment approaches would ultimately prove attractive to participating hospitals.

Thus, the longer-run effects of the Social Security Amendments of 1983 would provide rural hospitals with positive incentives to participate in the national swing-bed program. Nonetheless, only 149 hospitals were providing swing-bed care under the national program in December 1983. The fact that slightly over two-thirds of these hospitals were located in states participating in either the RWJF model program or the earlier HCFA demonstrations was evidence of the retrenchment brought about by TEFRA and the initial reaction to PPS. Less than 50 hospitals in rural communities throughout the United States had been willing to initiate, without prior experience, the steps necessary to undertake swing-bed care—a full three years after the enabling legislation. The RWJF model program, in conjunction with AHA-related activities, provided visibility for and information on swing-bed care, sustaining interest in the swing-bed approach during these early years.

A climate that was more conducive to innovation was introduced in July 1984 when the Deficit Reduction Act (DEFRA) was passed (P.L. 989-369). A new version of the dual Medicare reimbursement limits for hospital-based and freestanding SNF care was introduced, eliminating the single limit under TEFRA. Additional relief to some rural hospitals was provided under TEFRA by raising the PPS case-mix index for sole community providers. Roughly 25 percent of the swing-bed hospitals in 1984 and 1985 were estimated to be sole community providers of acute care in their geographic locations (under the Medicare definition for sole community provider). Raising the case-mix index, in effect, permitted higher per case Medicare reimbursement for such providers. The implications of shortened acute stays and the resultant need for near-acute long-term care were now becoming apparent since PPS had been in place for a reasonable length of time. At about this point, a substantial interest in swing-bed care took hold nationally, resulting in a growth spurt in the number of swing-bed hospitals.

Nonetheless, PPS brought with it a number of questions regarding the swing-bed approach. Paramount among these was the possibility that hospitals might game the PPS system. For example, if a patient was prematurely discharged from acute care, the hospital could theoretically collect its full per case reimbursement under PPS, admit the patient to long-term care in a swing bed, and still collect a per diem reimbursement for each day of swing-bed care. It could subsequently readmit the patient for another acute care hospital stay, thereby receiving reimbursement for another hospital stay upon discharge from this second hospitalization. This double-dipping phenomenon was theorized to be a potentially serious problem in swing-bed hospitals. Those concerned felt that rehospitalization rates for swing-bed hospitals would probably be substantially higher than for either non-swing-bed hospitals or nursing homes in rural communities. As a result, one of the major objectives of the evaluation of the national swing-bed program was to assess the extent to which double-dipping occurred. Rehospitalization rates for swing-bed patients would be analyzed, and the total cost of Medicare-covered services over a period of 12 months (i.e., longitudinally) would be compared for acute care patients admitted to swing-bed hospitals and patients admitted to non-swing-bed hospitals in rural communities.

Throughout the period from 1982 through 1986, a number of information dissemination activities continued. AHA held several regional conferences throughout the country for rural hospitals to learn more about swing-bed care. Speakers with experience in the swing-bed program were present at the various workshops, and a number of materials on implementing and maintaining the swing-bed approach at the hospital level were distributed. In addition, in February 1986, a swing-bed conference was held at the Brookings Institution in Washington, D.C. The conference was funded by RWJF and was intended to disseminate information on the swing-bed approach to policymakers and others associated with health care and long-term care (Wiener 1987).

Intensifying Case Mix in Hospitals and Long-Term Care Facilities

With the implementation of PPS, not only did acute care lengths of stay shorten in hospitals throughout the United States, but resource requirements for patients in acute care settings also intensified. Analysis of hospital case-mix and discharge data from abstracts submitted to the Commission on Professional and Hospital Activities showed that hospital patients generally required more acute care resources than had been the case previously. For example, while the average total length of stay decreased, the proportion of patient days spent in intensive care increased (Sloan, Morrisey, and Valvona 1988a). This increase in resource needs for patients was due to shortened stays resulting in greater per day service needs and the drop in the number of admissions to hospitals, presumably eliminating some of the cases whose care needs were less intense.

The change in case-mix intensity, however, was not restricted to hospitals. Nursing homes and home health agencies also felt the impacts of PPS and a changing health care environment in the early to mid-1980s. Traditional and chronic care nursing home patients were more dependent in functioning and activities of daily living than had been the case in the early 1980s. Medicare SNF patients tended to have more near-acute care requirements now than had been the case prior to PPS (Morrisey, Sloan, and Valvona 1988; Shaughnessy, Kramer, et al. 1985; Shaughnessy and Kramer 1990). Medicare home health patients were considerably more dependent in functioning by the mid- to late 1980s than had been the case in the first part of the decade, and also tended to have more near-acute care needs than previously (Shaughnessy and Kramer 1990; Guterman et al. 1988). Thus, the impacts of PPS and a general change in the nature of institutional care in the United States brought about a significant increase in case-mix intensity in hospitals, nursing homes, and home health agencies.

This changing climate in terms of care needs therefore circumscribed and defined the environment in which swing-bed care would evolve in the United States. At the same time that case mix was changing in small rural hospitals, occupancy rates were dropping even further in such hospitals, paralleling a national trend in occupancy occurring even in urban areas (Guterman et al. 1988; DesHarnais et al. 1987). Rural hospitals continued to have lower occupancy rates than metropolitan hospitals. Concurrently, Medicaid preadmission screening programs for nursing homes and the deinstitutionalization movement in long-term care were bringing about case-mix changes in traditional nursing homes (Shaughnessy and Kramer 1990; Lyles 1986). Despite the opposition of the nursing home industry to the swing-bed movement in particular, and hospital-based long-term care in general, a growing need for near-acute long-term care (fueled by PPS) was occurring. The manner in which swing-bed hospitals would respond was unknown but of critical importance in rural communities throughout the United States.

SWING-BED HOSPITAL PARTICIPATION AND USE OF THE NATIONAL PROGRAM

Hospital Participation

The growth in the number of certified swing-bed hospitals between December 1982 and August 1989 is shown in Figure 4.1. By late 1982, only 58 of the roughly 100 hospitals from the demonstration programs of the 1970s were participating in the national program. By the end of 1983, participation had increased to 149 hospitals. As mentioned earlier, however, of these 149 hospitals, 101 either had prior experience as HCFA demonstration hospitals in the 1970s or were part of the RWJF grant program. Despite the slow start, by August 1989, the number of certified hospitals had increased over 700 percent to 1,207 hospitals. The figures include hospitals certified as Medicare providers of swing-bed care, regardless of whether they actually provide long-term care in hospital swing beds. Utilization surveys conducted as part of the national evaluation study, however, indicated that approximately 97 percent of all certified hospitals were providing swing-bed care.

In addition to the number of certified hospitals, Figure 4.1 also shows the participation rates for each time period, based on the deter-

Figure 4.1   Number and Percent of the 2,236 Eligible Hospitals
Participating in the Swing-Bed Program from 1982
through 1989

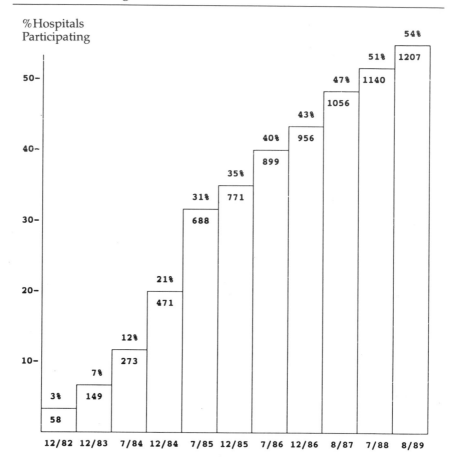

mination that 2,236 hospitals were eligible to participate in the swing-bed
program in 1984. In keeping with the 1982 regulations and subsequent
clarifications of those regulations, the Bureau of the Census' definition of
rural communities was used in determining eligible hospitals. A hospital
was considered eligible if it had fewer than 50 "effective" beds; in practice,
this means that a hospital may have more than 50 beds, but it is staffed for
less than 50. For estimation purposes in the evaluation study, the number
of eligible hospitals was determined by applying the annual occupancy
rate to the number of inpatient beds (a practice followed in some regions

to determine eligibility), exclusive of beds for newborns, beds in intensive care units, and long-term care beds, in keeping with the July 1982 regulations. The participation rates ranged from 2.6 percent of eligible hospitals at the end of 1982 to over 50 percent of the eligible hospitals by mid-1989. Due to hospital closures and changes in both the number of beds and hospital occupancy over time, the denominator for the participation rate doubtlessly changed over the time period covered by Figure 4.1. The rates should therefore be regarded as approximate.

We observed that hospitals with lower occupancy rates joined the program sooner, and as time went on, hospitals with higher occupancy rates tended to join the program in the later years. Nonetheless, a number of eligible hospitals still do not participate in the swing-bed program for a variety of reasons, including the perception, in many cases, that long-term care needs in their community are satisfied, or, in a few instances, that acute care occupancy rates are sufficiently high (a relatively rare phenomenon in rural hospitals) so that the swing-bed approach is not warranted. The August 1989 hospital count includes a few hospitals that in fact became eligible under an expanded swing-bed program (discussed in Chapter 7).

The relatively constrained growth in the number of swing-bed hospitals between 1982 and the end of 1983 appears due to the reasons discussed earlier. These include the delay in promulgating the regulations until July 1982, the negative effects of TEFRA later in 1982 on hospital incentives to innovate, and the implementation of PPS through the Social Security Amendments of 1983. Thereafter, the potential value of the swing-bed approach as a response to PPS, fostered by the information dissemination program sponsored by RWJF and AHA, served as a catalyst for a rapid increase in new hospitals participating in the swing-bed program.

The growth in the number of participating swing-bed hospitals was dramatic in the five states assisted by the RWJF program and in the four prior HCFA demonstration states. In the RWJF states, the growth between 1983 and 1986 was from 40 to 200 participating hospitals, a 400 percent increase. For the RWJF and HCFA demonstration states combined, the growth was from 101 to 400 hospitals (nearly 300 percent). The percentages of participating hospitals in July 1986 were 63 percent for the RWJF states, 57 percent for the RWJF and prior HCFA demonstration states combined, and 33 percent for all other states that had eligible swing-bed hospitals. Thus, it was apparent that the RWJF program helped several states get out of the blocks faster in implementing the swing-bed approach.

Figure 4.2 shows the geographic distribution by state of swing-bed

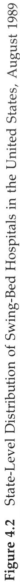

Figure 4.2   State-Level Distribution of Swing-Bed Hospitals in the United States, August 1989

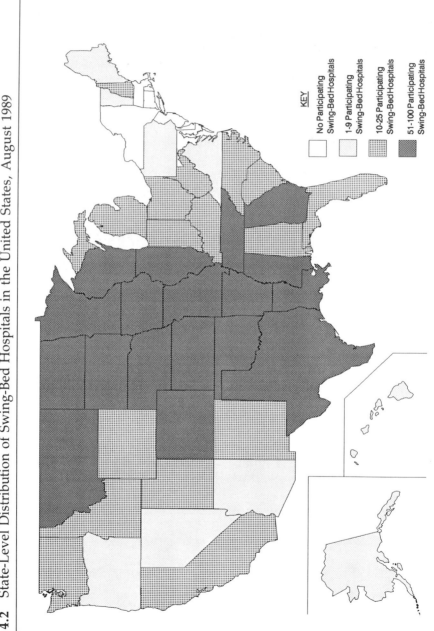

No Participating
Swing-Bed Hospitals

1-9 Participating
Swing-Bed Hospitals

10-25 Participating
Swing-Bed Hospitals

51-100 Participating
Swing-Bed Hospitals

hospitals in August 1989. The prevalence of swing beds in the Midwest is apparent. The large rural land areas that characterize such states are generally accompanied by a larger proportion of small rural hospitals than in other states, especially in the eastern United States. In fact, a number of northeastern states, such as Rhode Island, New Jersey, and Delaware, have no eligible hospitals and therefore cannot participate in the program. The relative paucity of swing-bed hospitals in the Northeast is therefore due largely to the small proportion of eligible hospitals in those states. In addition, certain other states, such as New York, had prohibited hospital swing beds either because of moratoria on long-term care beds or concerns about increased Medicaid costs. At this writing, New York State is implementing a modified swing-bed demonstration program for its small hospitals. Presently, Medicaid is participating as a payer in 20 to 25 states throughout the country.

Figures 4.3 and 4.4 depict the distribution of states according to participation rates in the national swing-bed program in 1986 and 1989. Unlike Figure 4.2, in these figures the shading by state corresponds to the percentage of eligible hospitals that are participating. These rates are based on the assumption that 2,236 hospitals were eligible for the program in 1986 and 1989. This is probably a slight overestimate in the number of eligible hospitals since some hospitals closed between the time of the initial estimate of eligible hospitals in 1983 and calendar year 1989. The rates are based on the ratio of the number of certified swing-bed hospitals divided by the actual number of eligible hospitals in each state. While there is a general tendency for states with greater numbers of swing-bed hospitals to have higher participation rates, there is not a one-to-one correspondence in this regard. As is evident from Figure 4.3, the nature of participation in the swing-bed program was characterized by an almost concentric pattern in 1986, with the strongest participation occurring in the upper midwestern United States. All states in this region had more than 50 percent of their eligible hospitals providing swing-bed care. An apparent, but somewhat less distinct, pattern characterized most of the states that bordered this region, with the majority of such states characterized by participation rates between 30 and 50 percent. As shown in Figure 4.4, this same pattern prevailed in 1989, although with more irregularities owing to increased participation in states located elsewhere in the country. Nonetheless, the program remained centered in the Midwest, where the swing-bed program began, owing in part to unmet demand for institutional long-term care in rural communities in these areas. Thus, the general participation pattern in the national program still reflects its origins.

The states with higher participation rates generally are characterized

Figure 4.3   State-Level Participation Rates for Swing-Bed Hospitals in the United States, July 1986

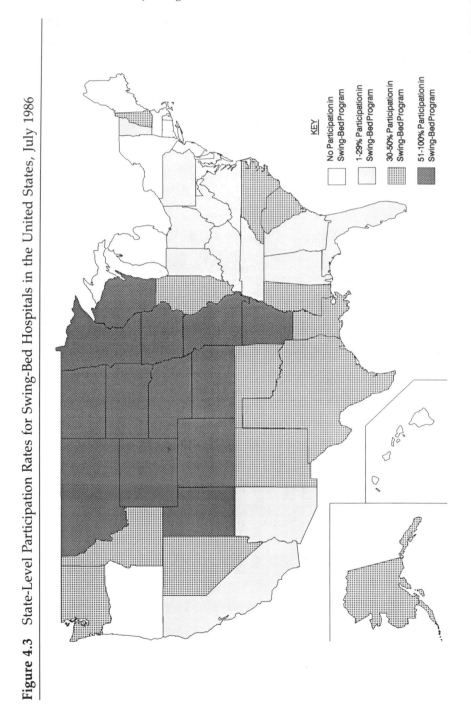

KEY

No Participation in Swing-Bed Program

1-29% Participation in Swing-Bed Program

30-50% Participation in Swing-Bed Program

51-100% Participation in Swing-Bed Program

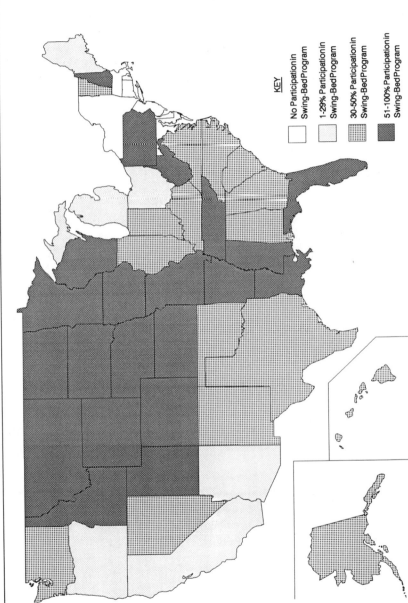

Figure 4.4 State-Level Participation Rates for Swing-Bed Hospitals in the United States, August 1989

KEY

No Participation in
Swing-Bed Program

1-29% Participation in
Swing-Bed Program

30-50% Participation in
Swing-Bed Program

51-100% Participation in
Swing-Bed Program

by Medicaid participation as well, although a few exceptions exist to the pattern of Medicaid involvement in states with relatively large numbers of swing-bed hospitals. Overall, we found hospital participation in the swing-bed program to be related to lower acute care occupancy rates, fewer acute care beds in the hospital, Medicaid participation as a payer of swing-bed care, a higher proportion of elderly residents in the county, fewer physicians per elderly in the county, and fewer Medicare SNF beds per elderly in the county.

Hospital Use of Swing Beds

The reasons cited by hospital administrators for joining the national swing-bed program were similar to those cited during the demonstration programs. The most frequently cited reasons were to provide better continuity of care, use staff more efficiently, provide additional long-term care alternatives in the community, increase hospital occupancy, use space more efficiently, and increase hospital revenue.

The average swing-bed hospital provided about 1,000 days of swing-bed care in 1985; of these, 49 percent were covered by Medicare, 8 percent by Medicaid, and 43 percent by private pay. The average length of stay for a swing-bed patient was approximately 20 days, while the average length of stay for a Medicare swing-bed patient was approximately 14 days. About 60 percent of all swing-bed days were SNF days (Shaughnessy, Schlenker, et al. 1989b).

Swing beds are often used as holding beds until long-term care patients are sufficiently rehabilitated to return home or until a nursing home bed becomes available in the community. Although about 9 percent of swing-bed hospitals provided more than 2,400 days of swing-bed care in 1985, most used swing beds to provide lesser amounts of care to near-acute long-term care patients (Shaughnessy, Schlenker, et al. 1989b).

The nursing home industry and others continued to express concern during the 1980s that swing beds were competing directly with nursing home beds. However, no statistical evidence of decreases in nursing home occupancy rates that were attributable to swing-bed care were found prior to 1986. An analysis of two states with a large number of swing-bed hospitals (Minnesota and Wisconsin) revealed no changes in nursing home occupancy in rural communities or, more specifically, even in swing-bed communities, from the year prior to swing-bed implementation until 1985. In fact, in Minnesota an increase in nursing home occupancy occurred in swing-bed communities over this period (Shaughnessy, Schlenker, et al. 1989b).

TYPES OF PATIENTS CARED FOR IN HOSPITAL SWING BEDS*

General Characteristics of Swing-Bed Patients versus Nursing Home Patients

Table 4.1 shows the differences between swing-bed patients and nursing home patients in terms of general characteristics. These findings are based on a 12-state random sample of long-term care patients who were in the 33 swing-bed hospitals and 40 nursing homes selected for sampling at the time of data collection. Swing-bed hospital patients were compared with nursing home patients (from certified nursing homes) in the same or similar communities. The difference in age between the two patient groups is inconsequential for practical purposes. The average nursing home patient's residence was more than two times as far from the nursing home as the average swing-bed patient's residence was from the swing-bed hospital. Thus, swing-bed patients tended to be treated closer to their homes than was the case for rural nursing home residents. A stronger home support system for swing-bed patients is suggested by the higher proportion of swing-bed patients who are married relative to nursing home patients.

The rehabilitation potential of swing-bed patients was found to be better than the rehabilitation potential for nursing home patients in the same communities. For over one-half of the swing-bed patients, rehabilitation potential was judged by providers as good or moderate; for approximately one-fourth, it was judged as good. This contrasts substantially with the corresponding 21 percent figure for nursing home patients. In keeping with the shorter stays just discussed, a higher proportion of swing-bed patients than nursing home patients had been in the facility for less than 30 days. This is consistent with the greater proportion of swing-bed patients classified at the skilled nursing level. The proportion of patients classified as skilled nursing care patients is somewhat imprecise since it involves using the level of care as determined by the provider (i.e., hospital or nursing home) and since the definition of SNF care varies from state to state. Nonetheless, it is informative because the magnitude of the difference clearly implies a stronger orientation toward near-acute care in swing-bed hospitals than in community nursing homes. This finding is further confirmed by the

---

*Selected material from this section is reprinted or paraphrased with the permission of The Brookings Institution from P. Shaughnessy, "Access and Case-Mix Patterns," in *Brookings Dialogues in Public Policy: Swing Beds, Assessing Flexible Health Care in Rural Communities*, ed. J. Wiener (Washington, D.C.: Brookings Institution, 1987), pp. 91–92.

Table 4.1   General Characteristics of Long-Term Care Patients in
Swing-Bed Hospitals and Nursing Homes, 1984 and 1985

Characteristics	Mean for Swing-Bed Hospital Patients	Mean for Nursing Home Patients
Age (years)	81.2	81.4
Distance to residence (miles)	20.8	49.9
Married (%)	29.4	17.3
Good-to-moderate rehabilitation potential (%)	54.3	21.1
Current stay less than 30 days (%)	55.6	8.1
Skilled nursing care classification (%)	60.1	37.3
Medicare primary payer (%)	46.4	8.7
Admitted from acute care (%)	75.9	50.8

Notes: Based on a cross-sectional sample (i.e., not an admission sample) of 552 patients in 33 swing-bed hospitals and 540 patients in 40 nursing homes. Mean differences are significant at the .001 level, except for age and distance to residence, which are significant at the .10 and .05 levels, respectively.

Source: Adapted with the permission of The Brookings Institution from Table 1 in P. Shaughnessy, "Access and Case-Mix Patterns," in *Brookings Dialogues in Public Policy: Swing Beds, Assessing Flexible Health Care in Rural Communities*, ed. J. Wiener (Washington, D.C.: Brookings Institution, 1987), pp. 92–93.

higher proportion of Medicare patients and patients admitted from acute care in swing-bed hospitals.

Case Mix in Swing-Bed Hospitals and Community Nursing Homes

The results in Table 4.2 are representative of results for a larger set of characteristics that were used to assess case mix in the national swing-bed program (Shaughnessy et al. 1989a, 1989b). The pattern of results for all such characteristics is portrayed by the representative findings in this table. In general, the case-mix results from the national program are consistent with those from the Texas, Iowa, and South Dakota demonstrations in the late 1970s. Further light was shed on the nature of swing-bed hospitals' tendency to admit more near-acute care patients by using indicators more reflective of patients' needs for such care.

The tendency of nursing home patients to be more functionally disabled is indicated by the findings for the first two categories of characteristics: patients with disabilities in traditional activities of daily living (ADLs), such as bathing, dressing, and grooming, and instrumental ADLs (IADLs), such as communication and housekeeping. Indicators of more severe disabilities in functioning were also analyzed, showing the general patterns evident in Table 4.2.

Table 4.2 Case-Mix Profiles of Long-Term Care Patients in Swing-Bed Hospitals and Nursing Homes, 1984 and 1985

Case-Mix Characteristics	Swing-Bed Hospital Patients	Nursing Home Patients
Percent with disability in activities of daily living (ADLs)		
Bathing	62.7%	69.1%
Dressing	60.1	66.2
Grooming	57.6	74.8
Percent with disability in instrumental activities of daily living (IADLs)		
Communication	14.7%	25.2%
Finances	58.8	72.5
Housekeeping	71.4	79.5
Laundry	75.6	83.7
Administering medications	60.1	84.2
Preparing meals	65.7	78.2
Telephone	30.8	42.4
Percent with medical or nursing problems		
Shortness of breath	20.5%	10.6%
Recovery from surgery	13.2	3.4
Intravenous catheter	6.3	0.6
Ostomy	2.9	1.1
Recent myocardial infarction with congestive heart failure	1.6	0.4
Catheter	20.9	9.3
Hip fracture in last 6 weeks	6.7	1.3
Stroke in last 6 months	7.3	2.7
End-stage disease	9.0	1.8
Urinary incontinence	34.0	48.1
Bowel incontinence	29.0	41.3
Mental status problems	40.3	58.9
Sociopathic behavior	8.4	18.3
Wandering behavior	6.9	10.6
Aggregate indicators (number per patient)		
Near-acute medical or nursing problems	1.2	0.7
Severe near-acute medical or nursing problems	0.5	0.3
Typical long-term care problems	1.7	2.5
Intense typical long-term care problems	0.9	1.6
General case-mix index		
Resource utilization group (RUG) index*	1.2	1.0

Notes: Based on a sample of 552 patients in 33 swing-bed hospitals and 540 patients in 40 nursing homes. Mean differences are all significant at the .001 level except for bathing, dressing, housekeeping, and wandering behavior, which are significant at the .05 level, and ostomy and recent myocardial infarction with congestive heart failure, which are significant at the .10 level.

*Based on an augmented sample of 596 swing-bed and 632 nursing home patients.

Source: Adapted with the permission of the Brookings Institution from Table 1 in P. Shaughnessy, "Access and Case-Mix Patterns," in *Brookings Dialogues in Public Policy: Swing Beds, Assessing Flexible Health Care in Rural Communities*, ed. J. Wiener (Washington, D.C.: Brookings Institution, 1987), pp. 92–93.

The third category of patient characteristics includes medical and nursing problems. Compared to patients in nursing homes, patients in swing-bed hospitals had a greater prevalence of near-acute and medically oriented problems such as shortness of breath, recovery from surgery, intravenous catheters, and ostomies. Although patients who had recent myocardial infarction with congestive heart failure were relatively few, such patients were found more often in swing-bed hospitals than in nursing homes. The prevalence rates for hip fracture and stroke support the pattern of a higher proportion of patients with near-acute needs in swing-bed hospitals. Specifically, greater proportions of hip fractures or strokes within the last six weeks or six months, respectively, were found among swing-bed patients. Conversely (but not shown in the table) greater proportions of patients with hip fractures more than six weeks ago, or strokes more than six months ago were found in nursing homes.

The more typical long-term care case-mix indicators corresponding to incontinence, cognitive functioning, and psychosocial problems exhibited a trend that was the opposite of the trend for the near-acute indicators. Higher proportions of nursing home patients had these types of problems, reinforcing the more traditional chronic care needs of nursing home patients relative to swing-bed patients.

The prevalence rates for severe near-acute medical or nursing problems, although not presented in Table 4.2, generally exhibited the same trend as those just discussed, with the exception that a slightly higher proportion of swing-bed patients had depressive symptoms. This was very likely attributable to the reactive depression that occurs following sudden traumatic events such as recent stroke or surgery, both of which were significantly more frequent among swing-bed patients. In addition, diagnoses such as fracture, major surgery, and neoplasms had higher prevalence rates for swing-bed patients, while mental disorders, circulatory problems, and nervous system disorders occurred with greater relative frequency among nursing home patients. The greater prevalence of circulatory problems among nursing home patients was due in part to past strokes, or to cerebrovascular or generalized arteriosclerosis.

Composite or aggregate scales for ADL, IADL, and medical or nursing problems were also constructed to provide summary indicators of the findings for these three general problem categories. The results for these scales further substantiated the pattern of a more near-acute care profile for swing-bed patients. This is demonstrated by the four aggregate indicators in Table 4.2. The number of near-acute problems and the number of severe near-acute medical or nursing problems were significantly higher among swing-bed patients than nursing home patients. Conversely, the number of typical long-term care problems, both in terms of prevalence and occurrence of more intense levels, was great-er for nursing home patients than swing-bed patients.

The final characteristic presented in Table 4.2 is an overall case-mix index based on an indicator used for Medicaid reimbursement for nurs-ing homes in New York State. The New York indicator was constructed by categorizing each patient into one of 16 unique resource utilization groups defined in terms of medical conditions and functional status (New York State Department of Health and Rensselaer Polytechnic In-stitute 1984). The 16 groups were constructed by dividing patients first into five clinical categories of special care, rehabilitation care, complex conditions, severe behavioral problems, and reduced physical function-ing. Within each of these five categories, patients were further sub-divided according to ADLs. The study data from the case-mix random sample of nursing home and swing-bed patients permitted an approx-imation of this grouping algorithm, with the results shown in Table 4.2.

The resulting index value is a reflection of staff resources con-sumed. The index, as originally constructed in New York State, was based on the nursing staff time needed for each of the 16 separate categories. The fact that the mean resource consumption indicator for swing-bed patients was slightly more than 20 percent higher than the mean for nursing home patients suggests that swing-bed patients are 20 percent more costly to care for than nursing home patients in terms of staff time required. This does not necessarily take into consideration, however, the different use patterns of certain types of ancillary services, such as diagnostic services and x-rays, for near-acute care patients and chronic care patients. Therefore, the 20 percent figure very likely repre-sents a lower bound on the extent to which swing-bed patients are more costly to care for than nursing home patients.

To assess whether the observed pattern of more intense medical and nursing needs of swing-bed patients might be due only to the great-er proportion of skilled nursing patients in swing beds, the same profile analyses were conducted using only SNF patients. This stratification lessened the number of differences between selected characteristics. However, the results of restricting the analyses only to SNF patients generally substantiated the overall pattern of greater medical intensity and skilled nursing needs on the part of swing-bed patients.

In summary, the results demonstrated a clear tendency for swing-bed patients to be more near-acute in their care needs. This was sup-ported not only by findings such as those in Table 4.2, but by consider-ably shorter lengths of stay, considerably higher proportions of Medi-care patients, and a greater prevalence of posthospital patients who were swing-bed patients. Thus, the near-acute nature of the care needs of swing-bed patients that had been suggested on the basis of the demonstration projects in Texas, Iowa, and South Dakota is now manifest nationally. The issue of whether swing-bed hospitals *should* be providing such care is an altogether different issue, however. Given the concerns about the quality of care raised in the demonstrations, this is no small matter. In fact, a major focal point of the evaluation study of the national swing-bed program involved the quality of care provided to swing-bed patients relative to nursing home patients. Its results would prove interesting and highly informative, carrying a lesson of serious import for structuring near-acute care policy at a national level.

CHAPTER 4 SUMMARY

Under Section 904 of the Omnibus Budget Reconciliation Act of 1980, over 2,200 hospitals in rural communities in the United States were eligible to participate in a national rural swing-bed program. Although some differences existed between the research recommendations from the late 1970s and the program as defined by the 1980 law and ensuing regulations, the parallels between the national program and the research recommendations were striking. It is important to emphasize, however, that a number of other factors coalesced, including industry support and the interest of both Congress and the administration, to shape the implementation of the national program.

The regulations for the national program were not issued until mid-1982, a fact that delayed program implementation. Before the regulations were issued, the Robert Wood Johnson Foundation (RWJF) undertook what proved to be an unusual yet effective endeavor to stimulate interest in the national swing-bed program. It sponsored a grant program that funded five state hospital associations and 26 hospitals in the five states to implement model approaches to, and information dissemination about, swing-bed care. Both by design and with some degree of good fortune, this program would eventually prove to be remarkably successful in accomplishing its mission. In late 1983, HCFA funded our research center to evaluate the national program in keeping with a congressional mandate to assess the viability and potential expansion of the swing-bed approach. RWJF funded our research center to conduct an accompanying study that focused largely on the quality of long-term care provided in hospital swing beds.

Despite the successes encountered in the demonstration programs and the enactment of federal enabling legislation, the new national program did not take hold quickly. In fact, between 1980 and 1983, serious reservations existed about whether many rural hospitals would undertake the provision of swing-bed care. In addition to the delay in finalizing the regulations, a number of changes in hospital reimbursement were introduced under the Tax Equity and Fiscal Responsibility Act (TEFRA) in September 1982. These changes, including a new rate-of-increase cap on hospital costs and elimination of separate limits for hospital-based and freestanding SNF care under Medicare, tended to stymie initiatives to innovate, especially on the part of small rural hospitals. Shortly thereafter, the Social Security Amendments of March 1983 implemented Medicare's new prospective payment system (PPS) for hospital reimbursement. The radical change from retrospective cost-based reimbursement, which employed the patient day as the unit for reimbursement, to prospective reimbursement, which used the case or stay, by diagnostic group, as the unit for reimbursement, was far reaching. It took a reasonable period of time for hospitals, especially small rural hospitals, to begin to sort out the incentives and disincentives under PPS.

By 1984, however, the climate for innovation by small rural hospitals began to change. Not only did it become clear that PPS offered incentives for rural hospitals to provide swing-bed care, but the Deficit Reduction Act (DEFRA), passed in July 1984, offered further encouragement. Modified dual limits for hospital-based and freestanding SNF care were reinstated. Some relief for rural hospitals under PPS was granted through the provision that roughly 25 percent of rural hospitals were judged to be sole community providers whose case-mix index (an index used under PPS to determine reimbursement) would be adjusted accordingly. Under this more positive reimbursement environment, greater interest in swing-bed care was manifest, although the incentives under PPS raised potentially serious concerns. For example, would it not be possible for swing-bed hospitals to admit an acute care patient under a particular diagnostic group, receive reimbursement upon discharge for that patient according to the diagnostic group, admit the patient to swing-bed care, be reimbursed on a per day basis for swing-bed care, receive reimbursement for additional ancillary services, and possibly readmit the patient to acute care under another diagnosis in order to receive per case reimbursement for yet another acute stay? It appeared that PPS offered incentives to swing-bed hospitals to shorten acute stays, capitalize on the per day payment for swing-bed care, and rehospitalize patients unnecessarily. HCFA augmented our evaluation study to examine issues such as these.

At the end of 1983, only 149 of the 2,236 eligible hospitals were participating in the national swing-bed program. Of these, 101 were either HCFA demonstration hospitals from the 1970s or RWJF grantee hospitals. By August 1989, however, the number of participating hospitals had increased over 700 percent to 1,207 hospitals, with more than half of the eligible hospitals in the United States participating in the national swing-bed program. What accounted for this growth spurt? Three major factors appeared to have come together to stimulate interest in, and implementation of, swing-bed care in rural hospitals throughout the country. First, after the smoke of confusion and policy change cleared, PPS offered obvious incentives rather than disincentives for rural hospitals to provide swing-bed care. Second, the RWJF model program implemented in 1982 allowed several hospital associations and hospitals to pave the way in dealing with patient care, reimbursement, certification, and information dissemination about their experiences. This both sustained the program in the early 1980s and provided the information base for its growth in the mid-1980s. Third, and perhaps most importantly, by the late 1980s, it became apparent that a genuine need existed for near-acute long-term care in many rural communities throughout our country. The swing-bed approach proved highly instrumental in meeting this need. The preponderance of swing-bed care was initially provided in the Midwest. Hospitals from these states remain significantly involved in the swing-bed program today. By 1989, only seven states were not participating in the national swing-bed program, all from the Northeast. Several of these had no eligible hospitals owing to the definition of rural hospitals under the national legislation enacted in 1980.

By 1985, the average swing-bed hospital was providing about 1,000 days of long-term care in hospital swing beds. Approximately 50 percent of this care was covered by Medicare, with only 8 percent covered by Medicaid. The remainder was covered predominantly by private pay. The average stay for all swing-bed patients was 20 days, with the average Medicare stay being only 14 days. It was apparent that hospitals throughout the country were providing primarily near-acute care in view of the high percentage of Medicare patients, the fact that over 75 percent of all swing-bed patients were admitted from acute care, the unusually short stays for long-term care patients, and the case-mix findings from the evaluation. Long-term care patients in hospital swing beds were less dependent than nursing home patients in functioning and traditional long-term care problems, but they were characterized by a greater prevalence of near-acute problems such as recovery from surgery, intravenous catheters, ostomies, shortness of breath, recent myocardial infarction with congestive heart failure, recent stroke, and recent hip fractures. Using an approximation of the case-mix approach for reimbursing nursing homes in New York State, the per day cost of care for swing-bed patients was found to be 20 percent higher than the per day cost of care for nursing home patients.

Although concern continued to be voiced by the nursing home industry, in mid-1985 no statistical effects of swing-bed care on nursing home occupancy were found. It was apparent that in rural communities swing-bed hospitals had gravitated predominantly toward providing near-acute care and were not competing with nursing homes for more traditional chronic care patients who required maintenance and palliative care. Key questions had to be addressed, however. Was the tendency to admit near-acute patients beneficial? Was the quality of care provided to near-acute long-term care patients in hospital swing beds such that it warranted continuing the national swing-bed program?

CHAPTER 5

Quality and Effectiveness of Swing-Bed Care in the United States

Since the quality of long-term care provided in hospital swing beds remains a critical policy issue unto itself, and since it also underlies several tenets in the final chapter, a reasonable amount of attention is devoted to conceptual, analytic, and empirical topics and findings on quality of care in this chapter. If the less technically inclined reader wishes to omit or skim through the more detailed presentations of the chapter, two options are possible. First, if a basic familiarity with the background and underpinnings of the quality-of-care analyses is desired, reading the first two sections (i.e., "Concerns Regarding Quality" and "Measuring Quality and Effectiveness") and the chapter summary would serve such a purpose. To simply obtain an overview of the basic findings and implications presented in the chapter, reading only the chapter summary should suffice.

CONCERNS REGARDING QUALITY

Quality of Care in Nursing Homes

Over the past two decades, quality of care and quality of life in nursing homes have been the focus of progressively increasing attention and concern (Kayser-Jones, Wiener, and Barbaccia 1989; U.S. GAO 1987; IOM 1986). As discussed in the first chapter, the genesis of nursing homes in the United States had paved the way for an attitude in the nineteenth century and early twentieth century that many of the predecessors of today's nursing homes were but warehouses for the infirm and chronically ill. Significant vestiges of this belief persist today. The belief was originally, and still remains, intertwined with the preposterous notion that residents of nursing homes somehow do not deserve, or at least need not receive, the care, respect, and attention warranted in other independent living settings and health care institutions, including good health care, a right to be as independent as possible, quality of life, and human dignity. Various exposés regarding nursing home care and abuses appeared in the 1960s and 1970s (e.g., Mendelson 1974; Townsend 1971). Several authors wrote about the problems we face as a society in terms of the quality of care and quality of life in nursing homes in the United States (Vladeck 1980; Moss and Halamandaris 1977; AFL-CIO 1977). Congressional investigations and hearings were held to examine these issues in nursing homes over the last two decades (U.S. Congress, House 1985; U.S. Congress, Senate 1974, 1984; U.S. GAO 1983; U.S. DHEW 1978). The work by Vladeck is particularly insightful in this regard; it traces events leading to—and reasons for—many nursing home problems that came to light in the 1970s. Although strides have been and are being taken to remedy problems related to the quality of care and quality of life in nursing homes, and although we have many good nursing homes in the United States, such problems not only persist, but remain widespread.

The Institute of Medicine (IOM) conducted a study in the mid-1980s to investigate and make recommendations about the problems that confront us concerning quality of care and quality of life in nursing homes (IOM 1986). Many of the recommendations from this study were incorporated into the Requirements for Long-Term Care Facilities enacted in the Omnibus Budget Reconciliation Act of 1987 (OBRA 1987, P.L. 100-203). The IOM study recommended that the Medicare and Medicaid standards for certification (i.e., conditions of participation) be strengthened and rendered more uniform. It advocated removing the distinction between skilled nursing facilities and intermediate care facilities for certification purposes. Emphasis was placed on uniform admission policies, regular assessments by registered nurses, adequate training for nurses' aides, residents' rights, quality of life, and access to patients for public officials. Outcome indicators and resident-centered surveys were recommended, using interviews and inspections. The report urged that regulation be based on the "performance of a facility in providing care rather than on its capability to perform. . . . There is a need to reorient the approach to regulation of nursing homes to make it more resident-centered and outcome-oriented" (IOM 1986, pp. 26–27).

The issue of adequacy of reimbursement may be related to quality-of-life and quality-of-care problems in nursing homes. Some feel that quality problems exist because reimbursement is inadequate (especially Medicaid reimbursement in some states). Others feel the relationship between quality and reimbursement is at best weak. No convincing empirical evidence has been put forth establishing a definitive relationship between reimbursement and quality of care to this point (Schlenker 1988). However, it would stand to reason that some reimbursement threshold exists, below which we should not venture lest the quality of care suffer. At the other extreme, there clearly must be a threshold point of no return or rapidly diminishing return with excessive reimbursement (Shaughnessy 1989). Realistically, however, excess reimbursement is not a problem in the nursing home field. It may be that our policies and practices have maintained nursing home reimbursement between these lower and upper threshold points—within an interval where the quality of care is little influenced by reimbursement amounts. It may also be, however, that the relatively crude measures of quality and the imprecise data analyzed to date simply have not permitted us to measure quality with sufficient sensitivity. This would perforce preclude an accurate assessment of the relationship between quality and reimbursement.

Quality of Care in Swing-Bed Hospitals

In Chapters 2 and 3, results were cited suggesting that swing-bed hospitals might provide worse care than nursing homes if a national swing-bed program were implemented. In view of the profound concerns about quality of care in nursing homes, if swing-bed hospitals across the country performed even worse than nursing homes, then the national swing-bed program should perhaps be eliminated. The quality-of-care component of the national evaluation was targeted at this question. At least one-third, and possibly as many as one-half, of all admissions to nursing homes in the United States are from hospitals (Kane and Matthias 1984). For some types of nursing homes, well over 50 percent of their admissions are from hospitals. Therefore, the point was stressed in Chapter 1 that hospital discharge is a pivotal entry point to the institutional long-term care system in our country.

This acute care portal to long-term care is at times characterized as much by disharmony and fragmentation as by integration. Although physician's orders are required to discharge from the hospital and admit to a nursing home, and although certain records typically accompany the patient from the hospital to a nursing home, thorough and comprehensive assessments of the long-term care needs of potential nursing home patients are infrequently done before hospital discharge. Assessments that occur shortly after nursing home admission are often inadequate. At times we are lacking in what should be concerted attempts to rehabilitate nursing home residents, especially shortly after admission, when rehabilitation care can sometimes make a substantial difference. When rehabilitation care is lacking for patients who have at least some rehabilitation potential, it is usually because of inadequate assessments or because of a prevailing philosophy of maintenance rather than rehabilitation that exists in many nursing homes. Patients are often readmitted to the hospital from nursing homes for emergent care, or diagnosis and assessment of problems that might warrant acute care. If the same emphasis that we place on assessment of acute care needs of patients were devoted to assessment of long-term care needs of patients, we would probably avoid many rehospitalizations, and many nursing home admissions from hospitals in the first place.

Of significant concern was whether long-term care provided in swing beds would be of inferior quality and possibly result in more rehospitalizations than might have occurred if the long-term care patients had been placed in nursing home beds instead of swing beds. Related to this, the previously mentioned incentives under PPS might encourage hospitals to shorten the initial hospital stay, still collecting the full Medicare payment for the stay; discharge the patient to swing-bed care and collect the per day payment for swing-bed routine care as well as additional ancillary care payments; and possibly readmit the patient to acute care thereafter, receiving Medicare reimbursement for yet another hospital stay. These concerns about the swing-bed approach were raised between 1983 and 1986. On the other hand, in view of the tendency for swing-bed hospitals to provide predominantly shorter-term long-term care, especially in the later demonstrations during the 1970s, perhaps they would focus predominantly on near-acute care under the national program. If this were to be the case, the more therapeutic and rehabilitative philosophy that characterizes acute care might prevail. It could result in at least average, if not above average, assessment and rehabilitative care for long-term care patients in swing beds. At the time, no one was even entertaining the possibility that we might be able to learn a great deal about providing near-acute care on the basis of the swing-bed experience.

Access to Near-Acute Care in Rural Communities

By the mid-1980s, in large part because of PPS, concern would surface regarding the need for and appropriate locus of "transitional" care. Initially, transitional care referred to health care needed shortly after hospital discharge in order to help in the transition from acute care either to institutional care to satisfy chronic care needs, or to home or some type of independent living environment. Various definitions and interpretations of the term *transitional care* came into play (Kramer, Shaughnessy, and Stiles 1989). Nonetheless, it stood to reason that long-term care provided in hospital swing beds might prove to be a useful and effective mechanism for transitional care for residents of rural communities.

The phrase *near-acute care* has been introduced in this book because of the multiplicity of meanings of the terms *subacute care* and *transitional care*. As used here, near-acute care refers to long-term care provided to satisfy the needs of long-term care patients requiring relatively intense medical or skilled nursing care, regardless of whether they were recently discharged from a hospital. They are usually at the higher end of the care-need spectrum for Medicare or Medicaid SNF patients. The term *subacute care* was originally intended to have this meaning, although it eventually was subject to a variety of different operational definitions in various states (Oregon Association of Hospitals 1986; Mitchell 1989). In some instances, the term *subacute* has been interpreted literally to mean any type of long-term care that is below acute care. For the most part, the term *transitional care* referred strictly to postacute long-term care provided immediately upon hospital discharge. Nonetheless, this phrase also took on different meanings in various locations and under different circumstances (Lewin/ICF 1988; Polich, Secord, and Parker 1986; Lipson and Thomas 1986).

Heightened awareness of the discrepancies in the health care delivery systems of rural versus urban communities has increased concerns that residents of rural areas are less likely to have access to adequate care and receive quality care than residents of urban communities (Coward and Cutler 1989; Moscovice 1989). This has led to several initiatives in recent years aimed at minimizing such discrepancies. For example, the federal government has provided assistance through the Rural Health Initiatives program, the National Health Service Corps and Area Health Education Centers, the Health for Underserved Rural Areas program, the Emergency Medical Services program, establishment of the Office of Rural Health within the Department of Health and Human Services, and the Rural Health Care Improvement program for augmented payments to rural hospitals. Other initiatives include funding of rural health care facilities by the Sears Roebuck Foundation, the W. K. Kellogg Foundation's Innovations in Ambulatory Primary Care program, and the Robert Wood Johnson Foundation's Rural Practice Project (DeFriese and Ricketts 1989; Moscovice 1989).

Generally speaking, residents of rural communities must travel longer distances to receive even emergency care, to say nothing of acute or institutional long-term care. Many rural communities in the United States that have a small hospital have but one or two physicians who admit patients to the hospital. Often, primary care physicians are the only practitioners of medical care in rural communities. If a person needs to visit another type of physician (e.g., urologist, neurologist), travel to a metropolitan area is required. Tertiary care and certain types of surgical procedures are available only in metropolitan areas. Especially in the 1970s and early 1980s, patients discharged from a rural hospital that required skilled nursing care or more medically oriented long-term care had to travel to metropolitan areas to receive these types of nursing home care. This particular access problem for long-term care patients has now been rectified in many rural communities by the swing-bed program. An even more serious difficulty in the case of rural long-term care patients is the distance family and friends have to travel to visit an urban nursing home. Since the support of family and friends is often critical to long-term care patients, especially those who have some potential for rehabilitation, this is no small matter (Brody 1986; Harel and Noelker 1978; Brody and Brody 1989; Dobrof and Litwak 1977; Tobin and Kulys 1980).

The demonstration programs in the 1970s had shown that the swing-bed approach clearly increased access to near-acute care for residents of rural communities. Considerably fewer patients, both proportionately and in absolute numbers, traveled to urban or more distant certified SNFs for near-acute care. Would this pattern persist for the national program? Although Congress enacted the national program on the basis of the success encountered in the four-state demonstration program, it was unknown whether these beneficial attributes of the demonstration would carry over to the national program.

The RWJF model program was intended to assist in this regard. The grantee hospital associations were to facilitate training hospital staff in their particular states and disseminate information regarding how the benefits of the swing-bed approach might best be attained at the hospital level. To the extent that the national program reflected enhanced access, hospital staff acceptance, moderate cost, and the patient satisfaction that had been attained in the 1970s, it would provide some measure of success of the RWJF program. Another indicator of success of the RWJF undertaking would be the degree to which the grantee hospitals in the RWJF program were able to "grease the skids" for overcoming impediments and problems that hospitals in other locations would encounter. Most hospitals that participated in the demonstrations in 1979 cited enhanced access and increased community retention of elderly patients requiring long-term care as their primary reason for providing swing-bed care. If this were to be replicated across the country, it would serve in no small way as a measure of success for the entire national program.

MEASURING QUALITY AND EFFECTIVENESS*

General Issues

Research on quality of care and quality of life in the long-term care field is presently receiving considerable and justifiable attention. Even for chronic or traditional long-term care, where outcomes can be difficult to specify and measure, concerns regarding quality of care and quality of life have stimulated a strong interest in analyzing patient outcomes. The interest in patient outcomes is well-founded, of course, since health care is provided with the fundamental intent of improving, maintaining, or constructively managing patient health status. Thus, influencing outcomes constitutes the raison d'être of health care.

That quality of care is characterized by a number of dimensions and viewpoints is well established and documented (Donabedian 1980, 1982, 1985). Although quality of care should ideally be measured through patient outcomes, attributing patient outcomes to treatments or care provided is far from straightforward. Mitigating circumstances and risk factors quite apart from treatments can influence patient outcomes. For example, a patient's ability to improve in ambulating after a stroke can be influenced by age, presence of skin ulcers, need for an IV catheter, and the extent of upper and lower limb impairment from the stroke.

The problem of attributing outcomes to treatments is exacerbated in the long-term care field, where pertinent outcomes often occur over relatively extended periods of time. Improvement in health status is often neither possible nor appropriate to expect for long-term care patients. At times, the most desirable outcomes include maintaining function, slowing the rate of regression of certain chronic problems, or minimizing pain and discomfort prior to death. Yet, at the other extreme, where rehabilitation is possible, outcomes related to improvement in function, and restoration to normal living, are expected. Despite recent and ongoing work to use outcomes in the long-term care field (Kane et al. 1983; Mitchell 1978; Shaughnessy, Kramer, et al. 1987), no comprehensive approach to assessing outcomes has emerged. Characteristics of the provider environment, termed *structural measures* (e.g., presence of physical therapy equipment, availability of x-ray facilities, adequate handrails for impaired patients), and services provided,

---

*Selected material in this section and the following section is reprinted or paraphrased with the permission of the Hospital Research and Educational Trust from P. Shaughnessy, R. Schlenker, and A. Kramer, "Quality of Long-Term Care in Nursing Homes and Swing-Bed Hospitals," *Health Services Research* 25, no. 1 (pt. 1, 1990): 65–96.

termed *process measures* (e.g., frequency of physical therapy provided to certain types of patients, number of physician visits, degree to which vital signs are monitored), are therefore useful in gauging the quality of long-term care (Kurowski and Shaughnessy 1983).

We have a number of regulatory programs in place at the present time to attempt to monitor and assure the quality of long-term care. As an illustration, federal peer review organizations were established in conjunction with the new prospective payment system for purposes of monitoring care provided (ProPAC 1986). Their quality assurance function for long-term care, however, is far from comprehensively developed at this writing. Certification agencies survey nursing homes and home health agencies on an annual basis to make certain that selected minimal standards (in terms of facility characteristics, staffing, patients' rights, and so on), are met prior to receiving Medicare and Medicaid reimbursement. However, none of these programs currently monitor outcomes of care or even processes of care in depth (IOM 1986; Lohr and Schroeder 1990). The grave concerns we have about quality of care in long-term care settings remain and will very likely continue for many years to come.

Measuring Outcomes: General Points

Considered rigorously, patient status outcomes are defined as *changes* in health status *between* two time points. The same patient status characteristics or variables used to reflect care needs for a given patient (or case mix across groups of patients) at a point in time can be used to measure outcomes between two time points. Further, in analyzing the change between two time points in a patient's ability to feed himself or herself, for example, other factors must be considered. In particular, patient status or case-mix factors (also termed *risk factors*) that initially characterize the patient, including the baseline level of the feeding disability, must be taken into consideration to properly assess the actual change in feeding ability between two time points. Such factors form a profile that determines or approximates patient prognosis for specific outcomes.

Single health status indicators (e.g., severity of decubitus ulcers, dependence in feeding) can be used to assess outcomes in a solitary or univariate sense. However, a patient is in fact a composite or constellation of health status indicators (e.g., feeding ability, ability to ambulate, skin condition, pulmonary condition, presence or absence of neoplasm, and condition of a surgical wound if present). Theoretically speaking, all health status indicators should be taken into consideration and measured simultaneously to properly assess patient status. Or, when measuring patient outcomes, such measures should all be considered simultaneously at two different points in time.

Therefore, when conceptualizing a patient's health status at a given point in time, it is appropriate to think of that patient as a set of composite observations or values on health status measures—some measured as dichotomies (e.g., presence versus absence of a surgical wound), some measured on an ordinal scale (e.g., a scale of several values reflecting the patient's ability to ambulate), and others measured on a continuous scale (e.g., diastolic blood pressure measured in mm Hg). It would be ideal if we were somehow able to distill this entire set of measures to a single measure that, when examined over time, captures total patient change over the period of interest. However, this is not possible, and we must typically settle for approximations or selected outcome measures. From this viewpoint, the analysis of a larger number of patient outcome measures is more desirable than analyzing a few, since such an approach would tend to involve more dimensions of individual health status.

Quality of health care can be measured in an absolute or in a comparative sense. To measure quality in an absolute sense, that is, relative to the way a caregiver "ought" to be providing care, expert opinion–derived norms that can be used as standards are necessary. At this stage, we are far from such standards in many aspects of health care, including long-term care. For the patient status outcome measures examined in the quality component of the national swing-bed evaluation, even statistical norms based on the manner in which long-term care is presently provided are not available. Consequently, a comparative approach of assessing outcomes for swing-bed patients relative to outcomes for nursing home patients was used. Adjusting for factors that could influence outcomes was important, especially because patients receiving long-term care in hospital swing-beds were known to differ from nursing home patients in the same communities by virtue of their near-acute care needs (i.e., their prognoses differ).

No single study can possibly examine the numerous dimensions of the quality of long-term care. However, efforts were made in evaluating the quality of swing-bed care to advance the state of quality measurement and analysis by comparing nursing home care and swing-bed care using a wide array of quality measures that are pertinent to institutional long-term care. The most significant quality results pertain to change in patient functioning, changes in the status of certain types of long-term care problems, and subsequent use of health care services. Various social, emotional, and cognitive attributes of patients were also examined to assess selected outcome differences between nursing home and swing-bed patients. Findings in the social, emotional, and cognitive domains of patient status were not as informative as the others, possibly because of less reliable data to measure patient conditions in these areas.

In measuring outcomes, not only is it important to consider patient status change between an initial and a final time point, but also the manner in which patient status fluctuates between these two time points can be important. For example, in measuring outcomes for decubitus ulcers, an improvement measured strictly between admission and the sixth week after admission can be misleading if the patient's skin condition changes substantially between the two time points. In a patient prone to skin condition problems, even though the condition of his or her decubitus ulcers may be unchanged at the sixth week relative to admission, improper care during the first weeks could have led to serious deterioration in skin condition. This might have resulted in stage III or stage IV pressure ulcers shortly after admission, prior to prompting more intense skilled nursing and medical treatment of the skin condition in the fifth and sixth weeks. Thus, in addition to simply assessing change between two time points, the stability of change or fluctuations in the patient's condition at interim time points should ideally be monitored when measuring patient outcomes. For this reason, patterns of change, including stabilization of patient condition over time, were an important component of outcome measurement in assessing the quality of swing-bed care nationally.

Using Care Provided and the Care Environment to Measure Quality

Providing appropriate services in an appropriate environment (in terms of staff, facilities, and equipment) does not necessarily ensure high quality of care in terms of patient outcomes. Nevertheless, health care delivery is premised on a presumed linkage between the process of providing services and influencing the course of a patient's condition or outcomes. In the acute care field, for example, surgical removal of a malignant tumor is often expected to resolve a cancerous condition. Administration of a drug or medication (e.g., penicillin or digoxin) can result directly in an expected outcome (e.g., elimination of a bacterial infection or reduced shortness of breath on exertion for congestive heart failure (CHF) patients, respectively). In the long-term care field, the proper blend of assistance in eating and encouraging the patient to feed himself or herself can result in the desired outcome of independence in eating. A well-administered bladder-training program or physical therapy program can produce the desired effect of a stroke patient regaining bladder control or independence in mobility.

It can be informative to measure the quality of care as reflected by the appropriateness of services provided to a patient (using data collected on services). This can be done by comparing treatment regimens with accepted standards for care in specific areas. Such analyses can be conducted under the presumption that well-provided services should produce desired outcomes, without directly measuring patient outcomes. This approach to assessing service provision for certain types of problems can be useful in the long-term care field, especially when outcomes, such as improvement in patient condition for chronic care patients, are not expected or are difficult to specify (or data cannot be collected on the outcomes). Therefore, measures of the processes of care or service provision were used in addition to outcome measures in assessing the quality of care in the national swing-bed evaluation study.

Certain attributes of the care environment can be regarded as necessary but not sufficient conditions for providing quality care. For example, regulatory standards such as those discussed earlier are premised on the assumption that staff capabilities (e.g., the presence of an RN supervisor or the presence of rehabilitation specialists such as physical therapists) and the availability of space for patient activities are necessary to provide adequate care. As a result, structural measures, or measures of the capacity of a facility to provide care, were used, albeit minimally, to measure quality of care in the national evaluation.

Adjusting Quality Measures for Risk Factors or Mitigating Characteristics

If desired patient outcomes are not attained, one of two basic reasons, or possibly both simultaneously, can account for the apparent failure. First, services may have been improperly provided, either by providing the wrong services (including no services at all) or by improperly providing the correct services. For example, providing services too frequently or infrequently, using an inexperienced or incapable provider, or being unaware of other services or medications the patient is receiving might negatively influence outcomes. Second, mitigating characteristics inherent in the patient or the patient's environment can influence outcomes apart from the services (e.g., age, diabetes, sensory deficit, neurological disorder, cognitive impairment). Since quality assessment or evaluation is targeted at determining the efficacy of services, the objective is to attribute failure or success to the service regimen (the first reason), somehow taking into consideration or adjusting for the concomitant or mitigating circumstances associated with the second reason.

Hence, in our study to assess quality of swing-bed care, it was necessary to adjust for risk factors or other circumstances that could influence quality of care apart from the health care provided. No pretense is made that we considered all possible dimensions of the quality of long-term care, nor that the totality of risk factors necessary to properly adjust all quality measures for mitigating variables were available. However, several hundred patient characteristics and risk factors were used in the context of measuring quality and adjusting quality measures for concomitant factors. In drawing inferences about the quality of care for swing-bed patients relative to nursing home patients, we therefore diligently attempted to compensate for any differences in health status and prognosis between the two patient groups. Overall trends and patterns in quality measures, rather than results for individual measures, were emphasized in reaching conclusions about the quality of care provided under the national swing-bed program. Details on the technical, clinical, and statistical aspects of quality measures analyzed are available elsewhere (Shaughnessy, Schlenker, et al. 1989b). Although sample descriptions are presented as needed in the next section, this reference contains further information on the various random and stratified admission, discharge, and cross-sectional samples used in the analyses whose results are summarized in the rest of this chapter.

QUALITY AND EFFECTIVENESS OF SWING-BED CARE

Patient Outcome Results

Findings on Utilization Outcomes. A prospective longitudinal admission sample of swing-bed patients and nursing home patients who were followed weekly for up to six weeks after admission permitted a detailed analysis of length of stay until discharged home. The stratified sample used for this analysis consisted of patients with at least one of four problems: confusion, incontinence, stroke, or hip fracture. The distributional curves (formally termed *survival curves*) for hip fracture patients presented in Figure 5.1 are illustrative of the results obtained separately for each of the other three problems areas. The two graphs on the left hand side of the figure pertain to all patients combined for the stratified sample, exclusive of patients who died. The two graphs on the right pertain to all hip fracture patients, exclusive of those who died. In reviewing the results, two points are noteworthy. First, the total-patients group is a representative sample of swing-bed and nursing home patients that have at least one of the aforementioned problems. Therefore, this sample does not comprise a random sample of all swing-bed and nursing home patients, but it is representative in the sense that these four problem areas are common in both chronic and near-acute long-term care settings. Second, the longitudinal nature of this sample corresponds to a relatively brief period of time, approximately six weeks after admission. The precise extent to which patients discharged home were subsequently readmitted to nursing homes, swing beds, or hospitals was unknown for these particular patients. However, for two additional samples of patients followed prospectively for six months after admission and six months after discharge, long-term care admission and hospitalization rates *after* discharge to home were not significantly different for swing-bed and nursing home patients.

The discharge-to-home curves in Figure 5.1 represent the cumulative proportion of patients discharged home at any particular point in time. Therefore, the higher the curve, the more desirable the outcome from the viewpoint of discharge home. As is apparent from the unadjusted curves, swing-bed hospitals generally tended to discharge patients home sooner and more frequently than nursing homes. This pattern is evident both for the total sample and for hip fracture patients. Although not presented as a figure, this pattern also persisted for each of the other three problem areas (i.e., confused patients, incontinent patients, and stroke patients). The discharge-to-home curves differ substantially primarily because a higher proportion of swing-bed patients are discharged home than of nursing home patients and not because there is a substantial difference in length of stay until discharge home between the two patient types.

However, the case-mix or risk factor differences between swing-bed patients and nursing home patients were substantial, as noted in Chapter 4. Therefore, the extent to which the differences in the unadjusted curves might be due to case mix was investigated further. The lower two sets of curves in Figure 5.1 represent case mix–adjusted (i.e., risk factor–adjusted—the terms *risk factor* and *case-mix factor* are used interchangeably in this chapter) discharge-to-home curves. Although the distance between the original curves was lessened through risk factor adjustment, it is apparent (and statistically significant) that, even after adjusting for case-mix differences, the cumulative proportion of patients discharged home (as a function of time) is greater for swing-bed than for nursing home patients. The same results persisted for the confusion, incontinence, and stroke cohorts in this six-week longitudinal admission sample. The characteristics/variables used to adjust the discharge-to-home curves for these various cohorts included not only case-mix variables, but also, in this particular case, the social support system available at home. The adjustment methods for the discharge-to-home curves entailed examining a number of characteristics as potential risk factors that could influence or mitigate the length of stay until dis-

Figure 5.1 A Comparison of Swing-Bed and Nursing Home Patients: Unadjusted and Risk Factor–Adjusted Cumulative Distributions of Stays until Discharge Home during the First Six Weeks after Admission, for All Patients and Hip Fracture Patients

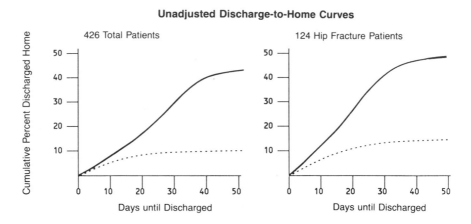

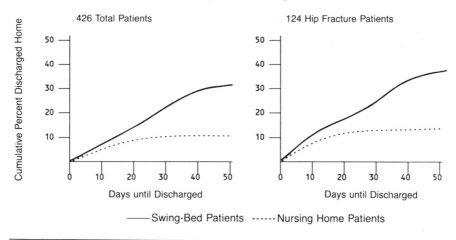

Notes: Based on 211 swing-bed and 215 nursing home patients in a six-week stratified admission sample of patients followed weekly for six weeks. All pairs of curves presented here are significantly different for $p < .001$. Patients discharged due to death were excluded from these analyses. The risk factor adjustments involved placing swing-bed patients at mean values for nursing home patients, thereby approximating the discharge-to-home curves (i.e., length of stay until discharge home curves) for swing-bed patients as if they had the same risk factors as nursing home patients. A large number of risk factors were analyzed using a stepwise survival analysis method. The variables given below are the only ones that were significant at $p < .20$.

charge home. Three of these case-mix factors were significant risk factors for the total sample, and four were significant for the sample of patients with hip fractures.

The curative or rehabilitative philosophy that characterizes acute care is very likely the basis for a significantly greater tendency for swing-bed hospitals to discharge long-term care patients to an independent living situation more frequently than nursing homes. This appears to be beneficial both from the viewpoint of enhancement of quality of life and cost containment. Additional analyses of case mix–adjusted patient outcomes were conducted to further test this hypothesis, however.

The distributional curves in Figure 5.2 pertain to the cumulative percent of patients hospitalized in two other prospective longitudinal samples. The first sample, the six-month longitudinal admission stratified sample, was structured the same as the six-week longitudinal admission stratified sample just discussed, except patients were followed monthly for six months after admission to long-term care in a swing-bed hospital or a nursing home, rather than weekly for six weeks. The four strata patient cohorts were the same. The second sample used in Figure 5.2 consisted of a random sample of patients discharged from long-term care in swing-bed hospitals or community nursing homes; these patients were also followed monthly for six months. The patients in the six-month longitudinal admission stratified sample were followed monthly for six months regardless of whether they were discharged. The hospitalization curves for patients in the admission sample therefore pertain to the first episode of hospitalization, which could occur any time within six months of admission, either while the patient was in the facility or after discharge. The hospitalization curves for the discharge sample pertain to the first episode of hospitalization, which could occur at time of discharge or any point within six months of discharge. Risk factor adjustment slightly increased the distance between the curves on the left, indicating that swing-bed patients tended to have characteristics that rendered them at greater risk of hospitalization than nursing home

---

The discharge-to-home curve for total patient sample was adjusted for three significant risk factors: (1) good rehabilitation potential, (2) an overall case-mix indicator based on the New York RUG-II system (see Table 4.1 in Chapter 4 and the accompanying narrative discussion), and (3) a bathing ADL scale.

The four risk factors used to adjust the discharge-to-home curve for hip fracture patients were (1) a scale denoting the patient's ability to administer his/her own medications, (2) a mobility scale, (3) a bathing scale, and (4) an overall index of ADLs.

Source: Adapted with the permission of Hospital Research and Educational Trust from Figure 2 in P. Shaughnessy, R. Schlenker, and A. Kramer, "Quality of Long-Term Care in Nursing Homes and Swing-Bed Hospitals," *Health Services Research* 25, no. 1 (pt. 1, 1990): 65–96.

Figure 5.2   A Comparison of Swing-Bed and Nursing Home Patients: Unadjusted and Risk Factor–Adjusted Cumulative Distributions of Times until Hospitalization during the First Six Months after Admission, and during the First Six Months after and Including Discharge

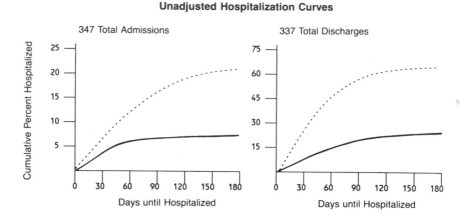

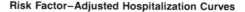

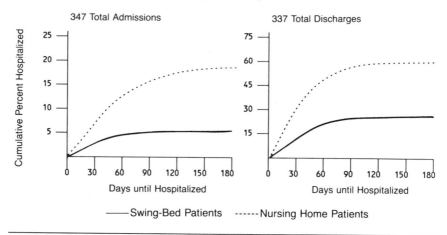

Notes: Based on 142 swing-bed and 205 nursing home patients in a six-month longitudinal stratified admission sample, and on 142 swing-bed patients and 195 nursing home patients in a six-month longitudinal random discharge sample. All pairs of curves presented here are significantly different for $p < .001$. Patients discharged due to death were included in these analyses, although mortality was tested as a covariate for risk factor adjustment. The results were basically the same, however, when analyses were conducted excluding patients who died. The risk factor adjustments involved placing swing-bed patients at mean values for nursing home patients, thereby approximating the hospitalization curves (i.e., length of stay until hospitalized) for swing-bed patients as if they had the patients—although other results clearly indicated that, regardless of this, such patients were not hospitalized as frequently. However, risk factor adjustment had little effect on the distance between the two curves on the right.

The fact that the pairs of risk factor–adjusted hospitalization curves for both samples are substantially different leads to two conclusions. First, nursing home patients tend to be hospitalized more frequently than swing-bed patients *within six months of admission*. Second, nursing home patients tend to be hospitalized more frequently than swing-bed patients *within six months of discharge*. In both instances, the conclusions are based on analyses that take risk factors for hospitalization into consideration. As already mentioned and to be discussed shortly, swing-bed patients generally receive considerably more physician visits during their institutional stay. Swing-bed hospitals also have more skilled nursing care available, which translates into greater attentiveness to monitoring vital signs and other patient conditions that, if regarded as unstable or problematic, might typically require hospital admission for a nursing home patient. In swing-bed hospitals, however, such patients are often not readmitted to acute care for further assessment. They simply receive the necessary assessment and diagnostic services as long-term care patients. Thus, a higher number of physician visits per week and more nursing staff who can treat medical and skilled nursing problems for swing-bed patients contribute to higher discharge rates to independent living, and to lower hospitalization and rehospitalization among swing-bed patients.

Survival Analytic Findings on Patient Status Outcomes. The curves presented in Figure 5.3 pertain to two different patient status outcomes for two separate samples. The unadjusted and adjusted curves on the left

---

same risk factors as nursing home patients. A large number of risk factor variables were analyzed using a stepwise survival analysis method. The variables given below are the only ones that were significant at $p < .20$.

The hospitalization curve for the total admission sample was adjusted for six significant risk factor variables: (1) a tube feeding disability scale, (2) digestive system disorders, (3) an indicator of maintenance-level stroke, (4) respiratory system disorders, (5) a meal preparation disability scale, and (6) an indication of whether the patient died in the six-month interval.

The four risk factors used to adjust the hospitalization curve for the discharge sample included (1) a toileting disability scale, (2) an indicator of urinary tract infection, (3) a dyspnea or shortness of breath scale, and (4) an indication of whether the patient died during the six-month interval.

Source: Adapted with the permission of Hospital Research and Educational Trust from Figure 3 in P. Shaughnessy, R. Schlenker, and A. Kramer, "Quality of Long-Term Care in Nursing Homes and Swing-Bed Hospitals," *Health Services Research* 25, no. 1 (pt. 1, 1990): 65–96.

Figure 5.3   A Comparison of Swing-Bed and Nursing Home Patients:
Unadjusted and Risk Factor–Adjusted Cumulative
Distributions of Stays until Improvement in ADL
Functioning (for Medicare Patients Only) and Improved
Toileting Ability, during the First Six Weeks after
Admission

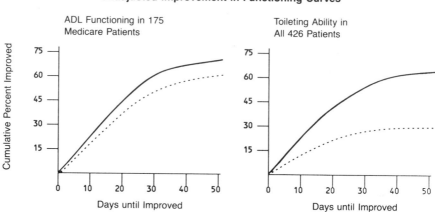

Unadjusted Improvement-in-Functioning Curves

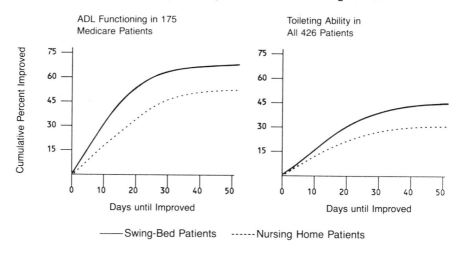

Risk Factor–Adjusted Improvement-in-Functioning Curves

———Swing-Bed Patients   ------Nursing Home Patients

Notes: Based on 211 swing-bed and 215 nursing home patients in a six-week longitudinal
stratified admission sample of patients followed weekly for six weeks after admission. The
pairs of curves are significantly different for the figure in the upper left at $p = .185$, in the
lower left at $p = .013$, in the upper right at $p < .001$, and in the lower right at $p = .019$.
Patients who died were included in these analyses, although mortality was tested as a

hand side of the figure depict the cumulative percent of swing-bed and nursing home patients that improved in ability to perform activities of daily living (ADL), as a function of time since admission. These analyses pertain exclusively to Medicare patients and are based on a discernable improvement in an overall ADL score index, the sum of six separate ADL dichotomies reflecting dependence (denoted by a one) or independence (denoted by a zero) in bathing, dressing, feeding, toileting, transferring, and ambulation. The difference between the unadjusted improvement curves was not statistically significant, demonstrating that, before risk factors are taken into consideration, Medicare swing-bed and nursing home patients improved at approximately the same rate over time in overall ADL functioning. However, after risk factor adjustment, the higher improvement curve for swing-bed patients indicates that Medicare swing-bed patients improve at a more rapid rate than Medicare nursing home patients in overall ADL functioning during the first six weeks after admission. The fact that the risk factor adjustment rendered the difference between the curves statistically significant shows that Medicare swing-bed patients, independently of care received (i.e., before care is received), tend to be at greater risk of not improving, or improving more slowly, than Medicare nursing home patients. Medicare patients only were used in this particular analysis as another form of case-mix control, since Medicare patients generally tend to be more near-acute in their care needs than non-Medicare patients.

The toileting ability scale associated with the survival curves on the right hand side of Figure 5.3 refers to the extent of assistance needed by the patient to get to and from a toilet or a bedside commode. As was also the case for the general ADL functional analysis just described, patients who were at the optimal state, that is, independent in toileting (or totally independent in ADLs in the case of the above analyses), were excluded

---

covariate for risk factor adjustment. The risk factor adjustments involved placing swing-bed patients at mean values for nursing home patients, thereby approximating improvement-in-functioning curves (i.e., length of stay until improved ADL functioning or improved toileting ability curves) for swing-bed patients as if they had the same risk factors as nursing home patients. A large number of risk factors were analyzed using a stepwise survival analysis method. The variables given below are the only ones that were significant at $p < .20$.

The improvement curve for ADL functioning in Medicare patients was adjusted for five significant risk factors: (1) good rehabilitation potential, (2) a recovery from surgery scale, (3) an intensity indicator for toileting disability, (4) an intensity indicator for disability in moving from supine to sitting, and (5) a communication disability scale.

The five risk factors used to adjust the improvement-in-toileting curve for all patients were (1) good rehabilitation potential, (2) an indicator of urinary incontinence, (3) a dressing ability prevalence indicator, (4) a toileting disability prevalence indicator, and (5) a communication disability prevalence indicator.

Figure 5.4   A Comparison of Swing-Bed and Nursing Home Patients:
Unadjusted and Risk Factor–Adjusted Cumulative
Distributions of Stays until Improvement in ADL
Functioning, during the First Six Months after Admission,
for All Patients and Hip Fracture Patients

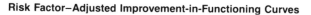

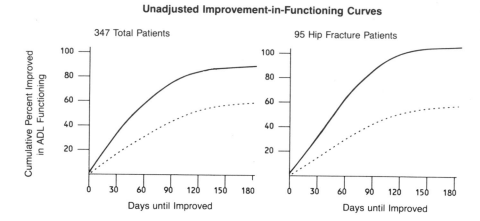

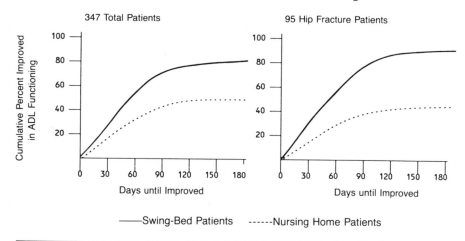

——Swing-Bed Patients   ------Nursing Home Patients

Notes: Based on 142 swing-bed and 205 nursing home patients in a six-month longitudinal stratified admission sample followed monthly for six months after admission. All pairs
of curves presented here are significantly different for $p < .001$. Patients discharged due to
death were included in these analyses, although mortality was tested as a covariate for risk
factor adjustment. The risk factor adjustments involved placing swing-bed patients at
mean values for nursing home patients, thereby approximating the improvement-in-
functioning curves (i.e., length of stay until improvement) for swing-bed patients as if they
had the same case mix as nursing home patients. A large number of risk factors were

from these analyses because they could not improve. This analysis included Medicare and non-Medicare patients together. The risk factor–adjusted survival curves for improvement in toileting ability after admission demonstrate a significant upward shift of the curve for swing-bed patients relative to nursing home patients. This suggests that the ability of patients to move from their bed to the toilet or bedside commode increased more rapidly in the six-week period after admission for swing-bed patients than for nursing home patients.

As with all other patient status outcome analyses conducted in the evaluation of quality of care, the multivalued toileting ability scale was first examined to ascertain whether there were different patterns of improvement (for swing-bed patients versus nursing home patients) according to the initial levels of toileting disability at admission. In those instances where differential patterns of this nature existed, the entire scale was not used; rather, patients were divided into subgroups for additional analyses. The patient status outcome analyses also took into consideration the length of stay until discharge for each patient. Thus, the survival analytic results on the lower right-hand side of Figure 5.3 reflect the enhanced toileting ability during the first six weeks for swing-bed patients relative to nursing home patients, after adjustment for risk factors and duration of stay.

Presented in Figure 5.4 are unadjusted and case mix–adjusted survival curves for improvement in ADL functioning for all patients (i.e., not just Medicare patients) and hip fracture patients, during the first six months after admission to either swing-bed care or nursing home care. The patient status outcome indicator used in these analyses was improvement in the overall ADL score index (the same as that used in the above analysis for Medicare patients only) representing the sum of six separate ADL dichotomies. The analyses were conducted for all patients

---

analyzed using a stepwise survival analysis method. The variables given below are the only ones that were significant at $p < .20$.

The improvement-in-functioning curve for the total patient sample was adjusted for seven significant risk factors: (1) good rehabilitation potential, (2) recovery from surgery scale, (3) an indicator of incontinence, (4) the baseline value for the Katz score ADL scale, (5) a toileting disability scale, (6) a mobility disability scale, and (7) a scale denoting disability in using the telephone.

The six risk factors used to adjust the improvement-in-functioning curve for hip fracture patients were (1) good rehabilitation potential, (2) a scale denoting the severity of skin ulcers, (3) a toileting disability scale, (4) an indicator of incontinence, (5) the baseline value for the Katz score ADL scale, and (6) a scale denoting disability in using the telephone.

Source: Adapted with the permission of Hospital Research and Educational Trust from Figure 1 in P. Shaughnessy, R. Schlenker, and A. Kramer, "Quality of Long-Term Care in Nursing Homes and Swing-Bed Hospitals," *Health Services Research* 25, no. 1 (pt. 1, 1990): 65–96.

pooled in the six-month longitudinal admission sample and separately for patients in each of four cohorts. The improvement curves in Figure 5.4 pertain to the all-patient and hip fracture patient analyses, although the results of the survival analyses for the additional three cohorts (confusion, incontinence, and stroke) were approximately the same as those depicted here.

In general, the results in this figure demonstrate that, after risk factor adjustment, swing-bed patients improved sooner and/or more frequently in ADL functioning than nursing home patients in the six-month interval after admission. Results similar to those shown in Figure 5.4 (for improvement in ADL functioning) were obtained for patients in other samples. It is apparent that most changes in functioning occur within the first three to four months after the initial time point.

The results in Figure 5.4 pertain to admission samples of patients followed for six months, some of whom were discharged and followed outside the facility. The attribution of postdischarge improvement or stabilization in patient condition to predischarge services is more tenuous than attributing in-facility change in patient status to care provided concurrently. This difficulty or tenuousness in assigning causality to patient outcomes is most pronounced for longitudinal discharge samples (the samples used in Figure 5.4 were longitudinal admission samples). A number of factors beyond the control of the provider can influence patient status outcomes after discharge, a fact that was kept in mind in interpreting results from the longitudinal discharge sample used in this evaluation. Tenuousness in assigning causality to patient outcomes is therefore less pronounced in the six-month longitudinal admission stratified sample, and even less problematic for the six-week longitudinal admission sample used in this study.

A number of survival analyses involving other patient outcome indicators were also undertaken. The general trend toward improved functional ability, after risk factor adjustment, on the part of swing-bed patients was evident in these analyses. Selected analyses for certain types of long-term care problems, such as incontinence, demonstrated the same general trend evident in Figures 5.3 and 5.4. Other analyses of improvement in skin ulcers, tissue fluid swelling, cognitive deficit, and urinary tract infections showed no difference between swing-bed patients and nursing home patients. The significant differences in survival curves tended to occur for ADLs and selected instrumental activities of daily living (IADLs), such as ability to prepare meals, and not in the cognitive, social, or emotional problem areas. (As mentioned, however, the health status indicators used to measure cognitive, social, and emotional disorders were not as reliable as those used for certain functional, medical, and skilled nursing long-term care problems.) In all, when differences persisted after risk factor adjustment, they demonstrated a uniform tendency for swing-bed patients to improve more frequently and/or more rapidly than nursing home patients.

It is possible and, at least for some outcomes, probable that the differences in cumulative proportions of patients improving in functioning between swing-bed patients and nursing home patients could be further reduced. In fact, some differences might be reduced to the point of insignificance with adjustment by additional risk factors more reflective of the chronicity of several of the functional disabilities (e.g., the patient's history). However, our interpretation of the empirical findings was also based on site visits, patient care observations, and discussions with a large number of physicians and nurses from the participating swing-bed hospitals and nursing homes. We therefore consider it highly doubtful that the observed differences could be totally eliminated through even more extensive risk factor adjustment. Rather, they demonstrate a substantial difference in the philosophy and efficacy of near-acute long-term care in the two settings.

Improvement and Stabilization Patterns for Findings on Patient Status Outcomes. A reasonably systematic analysis of patient status outcomes was also undertaken through the use of outcome pattern dichotomies relating to improvement and stabilization of patient conditions. Two outcome pattern dichotomies were constructed for a wide variety of different measures of patient health status. The first, termed the *improvement pattern dichotomy*, corresponded to a pattern of improvement of the patient condition by the final data collection point, with the additional requirement that the condition never worsened over the time interval from the initial point (e.g., admission) until the final follow-up point. The *stabilization pattern dichotomy* (nonworsening dichotomy) was similar, requiring that the patient condition at the final data collection point was no worse than the initial point, and that the patient's condition did not worsen over the entire time interval. For both the improvement and stabilization pattern dichotomies, a zero indicated that the specified improvement or nonworsening of the condition did not occur, while a one indicated it did occur.

Each such patient status outcome pattern dichotomy was adjusted for risk factors (using logistic regression). Case selection procedures to compensate for potential outcome differences due to nursing home and swing-bed patients starting at different levels of the patient status scale under consideration were used in a manner analogous to those used for the survival curve analyses just described. An initial or baseline value for the patient status indicator under consideration was also used as a potential adjustment variable or risk factor (as was done for the survival analyses). All logistic regression models (and survival analysis models) were developed on the basis of clinical considerations and then empirically tested using statistical methods. The Medicare-payer variable and mortality were systematically used as stratifiers and covariates (i.e., as sample delineators and risk factors appearing in the models). The results were always similar for these variables using both approaches.

Table 5.1 summarizes the results of the analyses of the improvement and stabilization outcome dichotomies. For each of the two longitudinal admission samples, the results of the improvement pattern dichotomies precede the results of the stabilization pattern dichotomies. The improvement and stabilization pattern results are based on weekly health status recordings for the six-week sample and monthly recordings for the six-month sample. The table contains neither all statistically significant findings nor all insignificant findings from the analyses. Rather, the results displayed in the table are intended to capture the general pattern of and typify the outcome differences and similarities between swing-bed and nursing home patients found in all such analyses.

The risk factor–adjusted results for the six-week longitudinal admission sample suggest that swing-bed patients tend to improve and stabilize more rapidly than nursing home patients according to several outcome dimensions. This pattern of more rapid improvement after risk factor adjustment on the part of swing-bed patients also substantiates the survival analysis results discussed in the preceding section. Since patients in this longitudinal sample were followed for six weeks, the improvement and stabilization pattern indicators necessarily reflects improved or stabilized condition over a relatively brief period of time. As mentioned, many of these analyses were conducted separately for Medicare and non-Medicare patients. In addition, Medicare was used as a covariate in those analyses where Medicare and non-Medicare patients were pooled (as in Table 5.1). Although the statistical significance of certain results, when restricted only to Medicare patients, diminished somewhat, largely due to smaller sample sizes, the overall trends and findings persisted for Medicare and non-Medicare patients separately.

The stabilization outcome pattern result on feeding ability for mildly impaired patients in the six-week longitudinal admission sample reflects the more refined case selection procedures discussed earlier; that is, it reflects the procedures used in addition to the general case selection procedure of excluding patients who could not improve or worsen from the improvement and worsening pattern analyses, respectively. Specifically, since swing-bed patients and nursing home patients were distributed differently according to their levels of impairment in feeding, and since different levels of dependency in feeding were associated with different rates of improvement and stabilization, mildly impaired patients were separated from severely impaired patients for this functional indicator in conducting the outcome analyses. Hence, the stabilization pattern results in Table 5.1 pertain only to mildly impaired patients for the six-week admission sample. Analogous case selection procedures were used in analyzing transferring ability for severely impaired patients and grooming ability for mildly impaired patients when examining the improvement pattern outcomes for the six-month admission sample in Table 5.1. (Since the improvement pattern results for both severely impaired and mildly impaired feeding ability were basically the same in the six-week admission sample, the improvement pattern results are not given separately for mildly and severely impaired patients in this sample.)

The risk factor–adjusted results for the six-month longitudinal admission sample demonstrated fewer differences between swing-bed and nursing home patients. This general pattern persisted for Medicare and non-Medicare patients separately. The fact that a larger number of unadjusted differences in outcome patterns became insignificant after risk factor adjustment for this sample than for the six-week sample may reflect a tendency for nursing home patients to improve and stabilize at a slower rate than swing-bed patients. However, it is also important to recall that a reasonably high proportion of patients in the six-month sample were discharged, with follow-up data collected while the patient was at home or in another care setting. Nevertheless, survival analytic results such as those presented in Figures 5.3 and 5.4 indicated that the level of independent functioning attained tended to be greater for swing-bed patients.

While not included in Table 5.1, the stabilization pattern indicator for decubitus ulcers yielded a risk factor–adjusted mean difference suggesting that decubitus ulcer problems stabilize more so for nursing home patients than swing-bed patients. The result was only of borderline statistical significance, but it was suggestive of better treatment of decubitus ulcers by nursing homes, a finding that was further investigated by assessing the quality of repositioning services for swing-bed patients relative to nursing home patients (these results are presented shortly).

Also not shown in Table 5.1 are the improvement and stabilization outcome pattern results for the six-month discharge sample. In general, the risk factor–adjusted differences for improvement pattern dichotomies indicated that swing-bed patients tended to improve more than nursing home patients after discharge. Conversely, the findings on risk factor–adjusted stabilization pattern dichotomies suggested that nursing home patients tended to stabilize more so than swing-bed patients during the six-month period after discharge. However, it is impor-

Table 5.1   Outcome Patterns of Patient Status Improvement and
Stabilization Adjusted for Risk Factors for Two
Longitudinal Samples

Six-Week Longitudinal Admission Sample

Outcome Pattern Indicator	Swing-Bed Hospital Mean (% Patients)	Nursing Home Mean (% Patients)
Improvement in		
Urinary incontinence	45.1	18.7
Mobility impairment	32.4	15.3
Bowel incontinence	33.5	14.0
Bathing ability	24.7	13.3
Overall ADL score	30.5	19.4
Feeding ability	28.5	18.0
Ability to transfer (NS)	24.9	19.7
Toileting ability (NS)	23.5	19.5
Stabilization of		
Tissue fluid swelling	80.6	59.6
Grooming ability	80.8	48.7
Overall ADL score	75.7	42.5
Social participation	96.2	64.0
Cognitive ability	79.8	59.8
Feeding ability for mildly impaired patients	78.6	64.1
Speech problems	76.0	65.7
Urinary incontinence (NS)	76.1	67.1
Ambulation (NS)	69.5	62.4
Bowel incontinence (NS)	77.4	69.3

Notes: Descriptions of the samples, including sample sizes, lengths of follow-up, and related information, are provided in both the text and preceding figures in this chapter. The same outcome measures do not (and should not) necessarily agree across the two samples because of the different nature of the samples, the different follow-up periods, and different patient locations at the various time points for the two samples.

The nursing home mean for each outcome pattern indicator is the unadjusted mean for nursing home patients. The swing-bed hospital mean was obtained by adding the risk factor–adjusted mean difference between swing-bed hospital patients and nursing home patients to the unadjusted mean for nursing home patients. This is tantamount to calculating the swing-bed mean after rendering the risk factor profile for swing-bed hospital patients the same as the analogous profile for nursing home patients.

The notation NS in parentheses next to an outcome measure indicates the mean dif-

tant to recall the aforementioned tenuousness of attributing changes in patient status six months after discharge to care provided before discharge. It is entirely plausible that outcome differences found for patients in the discharge sample might be eliminated by adjusting for other factors, including lifestyle and environmental characteristics after discharge.

Table 5.1   Continued

Six-Month Longitudinal Admission Sample

Outcome Pattern Indicator	Swing-Bed Hospital Mean (% Patients)	Nursing Home Mean (% Patients)
Improvement in		
Overall ADL score	34.0	22.6
Bowel incontinence	36.5	19.3
Ability to prepare meals	14.9	6.0
Transferring ability for severely impaired patients (NS)	30.5	15.5
Grooming ability for mildly impaired patients (NS)	17.4	12.9
Toileting (NS)	24.4	21.5
Stabilization of		
Tissue fluid swelling	89.3	62.3
Speech problems	84.2	68.9
Comprehension problems	90.3	75.8
Overall ADL score (NS)	51.9	40.0
Ability to use telephone (NS)	59.6	51.5
Bowel incontinence (NS)	72.6	68.5
Urinary incontinence for continent patients (NS)	70.3	67.2

ference is not statistically significant at the .10 level. All other mean differences are significant at the .05 level or less, except for improvement in overall ADL score and feeding ability for the six-week admission sample, which are significant between the .05 and .10 levels. In order to calculate the adjusted mean for swing-bed hospitals in the manner described above, the unadjusted mean difference was adjusted for risk factors using logistic regression. The statistical significance levels pertain to the significance of the odds ratio in a logistic regression model, with risk factors in the model.

Source: Adapted with the permission of Hospital Research and Educational Trust from Table 3 in P. Shaughnessy, R. Schlenker, and A. Kramer, "Quality of Long-Term Care in Nursing Homes and Swing-Bed Hospitals," *Health Services Research* 25, no. 1 (pt. 1, 1990): 65–96.

For this reason, the longitudinal discharge sample outcome pattern dichotomies that remained significant after risk factor adjustment were further adjusted for the location to which the patient was discharged.

In some of these supplemental analyses, using discharge to nursing home and discharge to hospital as additional covariates, the significant differences in outcomes between patients discharged from swing-bed hospitals and patients discharged from nursing homes disappeared. This may be an unfair adjustment process that begs the question, however. Poor care might result in hospitalization, for example, in which case it would be inappropriate to adjust for "hospital" as a covariate. Consequently, owing to the difficulty of attributing postdischarge outcomes to care provided before discharge, especially up to six months after discharge, the outcome pattern results on which our inferences are based are those obtained using the admission sample (and illustrated in Table 5.1).

Findings on Patient Outcomes Based on Percent Time in an Improved or Stabilized State. Outcome indicators corresponding to the percent time a patient was in an improved or stabilized condition also were compared for swing-bed and nursing home patients. As before, risk factor adjustment (based on multiple regression methods) and case selection were used in analyzing such outcome indicators. In general, the findings were consistent with those just mentioned. Swing-bed patients generally tended to spend greater proportions of time in improved or stabilized conditions during the six-week period after admission. Fewer differences between swing-bed and nursing home patients in the percent time in an improved or stabilized condition were found within the first six months after admission. In addition, swing-bed patients spent more time in an improved condition during the six-month period after discharge, and nursing home patients spent more time in a stabilized condition during the six-month period after discharge. These results were further substantiated by analyses of the change in status between the initial time point (i.e., admission for the two admission samples and discharge for the discharge sample) and follow-up time points.

Findings on Process Quality: Service Use

Descriptive Results on Frequencies for Selected Services. To assess the use of certain services, the relative frequencies of seven tracer services were analyzed using data from the case-mix random sample described in the preceding chapter (see Tables 4.1 and 4.2). The results comparing nursing home patients and swing-bed patients are presented in Table 5.2. They indicate that, relative to the average patient in certified nursing homes in rural communities, the average swing-bed patient had more physician visits, lab tests, x-rays, therapeutic antibiotics for urinary tract infections (UTI), prophylactic antibiotics for UTI, intravenous fluids, and intravenous medications. These are services that generally tend to be needed for more near-acute patients, reflecting the more intense

Table 5.2   Selected Service Use Profiles for Long-Term Care Patients in Swing-Bed Hospitals and Nursing Homes, 1984 and 1985

Service per Patient in Past Week	Mean for Swing-Bed Hospital Patients	Mean for Nursing Home Patients
Number of physician visits per week	2.8	0.3
Number of lab tests per week	1.4	0.3
Number of x-rays per week	0.2	0.0
Percent of patients on therapeutic antibiotics for urinary tract infection	5.3	1.5
Percent of patients on prophylactic antibiotics for urinary tract infection (NS)	7.8	5.4
Percent of patients on intravenous fluids	3.6	0.6
Percent of patients on intravenous medications	4.7	0.0

Notes: Based on a sample of 552 patients in 33 swing-bed hospitals and 540 patients in 40 nursing homes. Mean differences are significant at $p < .001$, except for the prophylactic antibiotic service for UTI, which was insignificant ($p > .10$)—denoted by (NS).

Source: Adapted with the permission of the Brookings Institution from Table 1 in P. Shaughnessy, "Access and Case-Mix Patterns," in *Brookings Dialogues in Public Policy: Swing Beds, Assessing Flexible Health Care in Rural Communities*, ed. J. Wiener (Washington, D.C.: Brookings Institution, 1987), pp. 92–93.

near-acute case mix of swing-bed hospitals. Risk factor adjustment of the mean differences in Table 5.2 was conducted using the approaches described in the preceding section. After adjustment, although not shown in Table 5.2, the mean differences between both therapeutic and prophylactic antibiotics for UTI, and for intravenous fluids, were insignificant. The significant adjusted differences between swing-bed hospitals and nursing homes for physician visits, lab tests, x-rays, and intravenous medications point to a difference in overall orientation of the two provider types.

From the viewpoint of resource consumption and potential overuse of services, these results suggest possible inefficiencies or lack of cost consciousness by swing-bed hospitals. However, from the viewpoint of quality of care, including accessibility to physician services, diagnostic services, and services provided by highly qualified nurses, this utilization pattern also suggests higher-quality near-acute care in swing-bed hospitals. Most importantly, the results involving patient status outcomes and utilization outcomes just described tend to substantiate that beneficial outcomes resulted from this service use. As discussed in the next chapter, this translates into a cost-effective approach (from the perspective of payers, including Medicare) to providing long-term care. Further, site visits and conversations with providers indicated that the frequency and use of such services led to avoiding hospitalization of swing-bed patients and earlier discharge to independent living environments—further supporting the findings described previously in this chapter.

The services presented in Table 5.2 were also compared for Robert Wood Johnson Foundation (RWJF) grantee hospitals relative to other swing-bed hospitals. After case-mix adjustment, three mean differences persisted. Unlike the insignificance of the difference between swing-bed hospital and nursing home patients in Table 5.2, a significantly higher percentage of patients on prophylactic antibiotics for urinary tract infection was found in RWJF grantee hospitals than other swing-bed hospitals. This finding was of some concern since it is not generally considered good care to administer prophylactic antibiotics to prevent urinary tract infections in susceptible patients; that is, it tends to fall in the category of overmedication. RWJF grantee hospital swing-bed patients were found to experience lower utilization of lab tests and x-rays than other swing-bed patients. This would seem to indicate a greater degree of efficiency on the part of the RWJF hospitals, without reducing effectiveness, since no substantial differences in the quality of care were found between the two facility types (except for the potential difficulty with prophylactic antibiotics).

Process Quality Comparisons. For each patient in the six-week longitudinal admission sample, data were collected on 27 separate long-term care services. The primary intent was to assess the quality of care provided to chronic care patients using process measures of quality. The services included largely those more typically provided in traditional long-term care settings. Some of the services, however, also were pertinent to the provision of near-acute care. They included assistance or therapeutic services in the following areas:

1. bathing	10. skin ulcer care
2. dressing	11. personal interaction
3. grooming	12. activity programs
4. eating	13. blood pressure
5. elimination	14. pressure relief
6. walking	15. pain control
7. transferring	16. range of motion
8. repositioning	17. physical therapy
9. preventive skin care	18. occupational therapy

19. speech therapy
20. reality orientation
21. environmental therapy
22. assistive devices
23. protective services for wandering

24. psychotherapy
25. catheterization
26. bladder training
27. devices for control of incontinence

For each service, data were collected on whether the service was provided in the past week, the frequency with which it was provided, and the provider(s) of the services. In addition, contraindications to service provision were also obtained through information collected on patient conditions. Thus, the nature of the sample and data collection permitted analyses of whether each of the 27 services was provided, the extent to which it was provided, and the provider of the service. Such data were available for patients stratified according to the four patient strata (discussed earlier) in the six-week longitudinal admission sample, with the ability to take into consideration whether individual patient conditions contraindicated provision of certain services. The incontinence, stroke, and hip fracture strata were further subdivided (into substrata) according to whether the nature of the patient's problem basically required maintenance services rather than rehabilitation services. The service provision data, taking contraindications into consideration, were then analyzed for the various strata and substrata, individually and combined.

In addition to purely descriptive statistics on service provision, process quality scores were constructed. They were based on, and represented refinements of, approaches used in previous studies (Shaughnessy, Breed, and Landes 1982). The services were identified and operationalized with the help of quality advisory panels consisting of multidisciplinary groups of experts in the long-term care field. The panels included registered nurses, physicians, physical therapists, social workers, and other researchers and practitioners. Numeric weights characterizing the appropriateness and importance of individual services for the specific problem cohorts were developed for use in the evaluation. Individual quality scores were computed for each service and then aggregated to the individual problem level (i.e., the problems that define the strata and substrata), both on a service-specific bias and for groups or clusters of services.

The effects of case-mix (risk factor) differences between swing-bed hospitals and nursing homes on differences in process quality scores were first assessed by separately analyzing patients according to the four strata (i.e., confused, incontinent, hip fracture, and stroke patients). Thereafter, case mix–adjusted analyses were conducted within strata and for all patients pooled. The case-mix adjustments involved treating each quality score as a dependent variable in a regression equation with independent variables consisting of case-mix variables and an indicator variable corresponding to whether each patient was a swing-bed or nursing home patient. The quality scores tended to be approximately normally distributed, rendering the regression approach acceptable from the viewpoint of the underlying distribution of the dependent variable. Other methods, including estimating regression equations for the nursing home patients and then substituting case-mix profiles for swing-bed patients into the nursing home regression equations were also employed, yielding approximately the same results as those described here.

After adjusting for case mix, the process quality results suggested that nursing homes were characterized by higher case mix–adjusted average quality scores in the areas of traditional ADL and nursing services (e.g., dressing, assistance with elimination, preventive skin care, repositioning, and social/recreational activities). The finding on repositioning reinforced the borderline result mentioned earlier, that nursing home patients had slightly better outcomes for decubitus ulcers than swing-bed patients. Overall, the results tended to be consistent with the earlier demonstration results, suggesting that "chronic care" services provided to more chronically ill or traditional nursing home patients in swing beds were less adequate than analogous care provided in nursing homes. Although a few of the findings suggested near-acute care services might be better provided in swing-bed hospitals, they were not pronounced, nor did the analysis include an adequate spectrum of such services to provide definitive evidence.

Since the approach taken to process quality measurement is strongly influenced by the frequency with which services are provided, two general caveats are appropriate. First, the provision of services in accordance with specified standards for frequency does not necessarily ensure positive outcomes. Since only selected services were used in this analysis, others that were not analyzed could have been equally or even more important in influencing outcomes (e.g., medications, physician care). Second, for various types of ADL and chronic care services especially, there is some concern in the long-term care field that dependency is promoted and even fostered by the overprovision of ADL services. As mentioned in the first chapter, since chronic care case mix in many nursing homes necessitates that aides (the typical providers of most services in nursing homes) be trained to routinely provide such services to most nursing home residents, the habit of providing such services can negate the tendency to encourage patients to function as independently as possible. This dependency-fostering approach to providing these services can result in what appears to be higher-quality care from a process perspective, but it does not necessarily result in improved patient status. In fact, it can result in declining functional status over time. Nonetheless, many nursing home patients cannot be expected to function independently, requiring that providers treat such patients as chronically ill and permanently debilitated in ADLs, urinary incontinence, bowel incontinence, and cognitive functioning. The fine line between adequate provision of services and overprovision of services to long-term care patients is, at times, difficult to discern.

Structural Quality

By the 1980s, it was evident that considerable variation existed from state to state in (1) the stringency with which SNF certification surveys were conducted and (2) the extent of sanctions associated with enforcing the SNF regulations (IOM 1986). Because of this, and because of the additional flexibility in regulatory requirements for swing-bed hospitals, the process of certifying swing beds for SNF care also varied from state to state. The regulations emphasized several areas (either conditions or standards in the SNF regulations) that should be required of swing-bed hospitals and that were not felt to impose a significant burden on rural hospitals. These areas included patients' rights, specialized rehabilitative services (referring primarily to physical therapy, speech therapy, and occupational therapy), dental services, social services, patient activities, and discharge planning. The SNF requirements of dining and patient activity rooms were not stringently enforced since, in some instances, this would require structural modifications for hospitals providing relatively small amounts of long-term care.

Site visits and discussions with certification agencies indicated that swing-bed hospitals tended to satisfy the patients' rights standard without any major problems. For patients in the longitudinal discharge samples, it was found that written discharge plans were more prevalent for swing-bed hospital patients than nursing home patients. Findings associated with the remaining areas of concern identified in the 1982 regulations are presented in Table 5.3.

This table presents the compliance rates for selected Medicare SNF conditions of participation (or required services) for swing-bed hospitals in 1978 and 1984, and for comparison SNFs in 1978. As reported earlier, swing-bed hospitals were notably deficient, relative to nursing homes, in meeting the conditions of participation during the 1978 demonstration programs in Texas, Iowa, and South Dakota. It is clear that a higher proportion of swing-bed patients were complying with these conditions of participation by 1984. Although on-site verification suggested that

Table 5.3   Percentage of Facilities Meeting Selected Conditions of
Participation by Type of Facility

	Compliance Rates by Facility		
SNF Condition of Participation	81 Demonstration Swing-Bed Hospitals in 1978	33 Comparison SNFs in 1978	55 Swing-Bed Hospitals in 1984
Physical therapy*	53%	100%	96%
Speech therapy*	17	58	56
Occupational therapy*	5	30	52
Dental services	52	94	98
Social services	36	97	98
Patient activities	16	97	93

Notes: Data obtained from both provider surveys for hospital administrators and Medicare/Medicaid skilled nursing facility survey reports. Differences between the 1978 demonstration hospitals and both the comparison SNFs and 1984 swing-bed hospitals are all significant at $p < .001$.

*These services do not refer to three separate SNF conditions of participation. Rather, they all fall under the specialized rehabilitation services condition. The facility is required to have such services available, either through its staff or a contractual arrangement, as needed by patients to improve and maintain function. A facility is not required to offer such services if it does not admit or retain patients who need them.

compliance rates for social services and patient activities may have been biased upward, it was evident that swing-bed hospitals were now in substantially greater compliance with the key conditions of participation than in the demonstration era.

The capacity of swing-bed hospitals to care for near-acute patients was further reinforced by the significantly higher proportion of ancillary services available in swing-bed hospitals (relative to nursing homes) directly through the facility's staff rather than through contracts with external providers in the areas of physical therapy, respiratory therapy, laboratory services, and x-ray services. Informal discussions held later in 1986 and 1987 suggested that more physical therapy was very likely being provided after the hospitals became familiar with the swing-bed approach than during their initial two years. Nursing homes had a significantly higher proportion of staff members involved in the direct provision of social services than swing-bed hospitals who contracted for such services (often from a local nursing home).

Surveys of directors of nursing in swing-bed hospitals and comparison nursing homes covered the issue of staff involvement in care planning and discharge planning. The most important statistically significant differences between swing-bed hospitals and comparison nursing homes in this regard entailed the involvement of dieticians, social workers, and activities directors in care planning. In swing-bed hospitals, dieticians were more frequently involved in care planning than in nursing homes, while social workers and activities directors were more frequently involved in nursing homes. Few differences existed in staff involvement in discharge planning. One noteworthy difference was that physicians were more involved in discharge planning for swing-bed patients than for nursing home patients, although the difference was not substantial.

Access and Community Retention

As indicated in Chapter 4, the most frequently cited reason by hospital administrators for joining the national swing-bed program was to provide better continuity of care for patients. The second most frequently cited reason was to use staff more efficiently, while the third was to provide better long-term care alternatives in the community. Surveys of directors of nursing and physicians in 1985 indicated that nearly all physicians felt that the swing-bed program resulted in more patients receiving long-term care in their home community than previously. By and large, nearly all directors of nursing of swing-bed hospitals felt the same, while approximately two-thirds of directors of nursing in community nursing homes agreed the swing-bed approach had enhanced community retention of long-term care patients. These findings were further supported by an analysis of Medicare claims data that showed considerably greater proportions of Medicare patients now receiving SNF care in swing-bed communities than had been the case prior to implementation of the swing-bed program.

FINAL POINTS

The empirical findings on quality of care and effectiveness of care under the swing-bed approach leave little doubt that swing-bed hospitals are providing higher-quality care to near-acute patients in rural communities than had been the case prior to the national swing-bed program. However, as in the demonstration projects in the 1970s, it also appears that nursing homes provide higher-quality care to long-term care patients in need of chronic care or traditional nursing home care. Since swing-bed hospitals have demonstrated a clear tendency to admit near-acute care patients rather than chronic care patients, this leads to the conclusion that swing-bed hospitals have been highly effective in providing care to the types of long-term care patients that they typically admit. The findings presented in the next chapter resulted from analyses targeted at the cost of such care. Considered in the context of the findings on quality of care, such analyses had the potential to lead to the conclusion that the swing-bed approach is a cost-effective means of providing near-acute care in rural communities.

CHAPTER 5 SUMMARY

Concerns about the quality of care and quality of life in our country's nursing homes have surfaced in a variety of ways during the past two decades. Without doubt, this is a critical public policy issue. Who is to blame for our quality-of-care problems and how they might be remedied systematically is beyond our purview here. But we do not want to make matters worse. If the quality of long-term care provided in hospital swing beds in the United States is worse than the quality of nursing home care, we would be doing just this. The question of whether quality under the swing-bed approach is at least comparable to the quality of long-term care provided in nursing homes is, therefore, an important issue not only from the perspective of the swing-bed program, but more broadly from the perspective of at least maintaining the quality of institutional long-term care in the United States. In framing our approach to analyzing quality, virtually no one expected we might actually learn how to improve long-term care by studying the fledgling swing-bed program.

When assessing the quality of care, a number of points must be taken into consideration. Generally speaking, it is not possible to comprehensively assess quality owing to its numerous dimensions. Most would agree that patient outcomes constitute the essential feature of quality of care; that is, we judge care to be successful if it brings about desired outcomes in patient well-being in areas such as physiologic improvement, maintenance of function, slowing regression of chronic problems, pain minimization, or even coping with death. Health services are critical because they are a means to attaining health care outcomes. However important it might be to examine service provision in assessing the quality of care, the manner in which services are provided cannot alone be a measure of the effectiveness of care—this is the purview of patient outcomes. Analogously, the structure of the care environment, including factors such as qualifications of providers, availability of equipment, and physical design of a facility, is important and can influence the quality of care, but in itself is not as accurate a gauge of quality as outcomes.

These three dimensions of quality—outcomes of care (e.g., reduced hospitalization and increased independence in functioning), processes of care (e.g., frequency of physician visits and lab services provided), and structure of the care environment (e.g., availability of physical therapy services and dental services)—can be translated into quantifiable measures that shed light on the quality of care provided. All three types of measures were used in the evaluation of the quality of long-term care provided in hospital swing beds relative to that provided in nursing homes. Another attribute of care related to quality is access. In this regard, the extent to which patients received long-term care in their home community before and after the national swing-bed program was analyzed in rural areas that had swing-bed hospitals. After the results were obtained, we asked physicians and nurses at the swing-bed hospitals and the nursing homes involved in the study whether they felt the research findings accurately reflected the nature of the care provided.

Patient outcomes were analyzed in two basic ways. First, *utilization outcomes,* which pertain to service use or nonuse after an episode of care, were employed. The two most important utilization outcomes were discharge to home and hospitalization after an episode of care. Second, different approaches were used to analyze *patient status outcomes,* or actual change in patient conditions over time. The time until a given condition (such as dependence in ambulation) improved was analyzed using statistical and graphical methods of survival analysis. These permitted a comparison of curves reflecting time until improvement for nursing home patients and swing-bed hospital patients. Another way patient status outcomes were analyzed was by constructing indicators of patterns of improvement or stabilization. For example, a patient was defined to exhibit a pattern of improvement (in dressing ability, say) if a disability scale showed improvement at a given time point after admission and never worsened thereafter. We also utilized time spent in an improved or stabilized state (relative to admission) as yet another way to compare patient status outcomes between nursing home patients and swing-bed patients. In all instances, we adjusted for case-mix or risk factor differences between nursing home patients and swing-bed patients. Since swing-bed patients were found to be more near-acute in their care needs than nursing home patients, who were found to have more chronic care needs, the statistical analyses controlled for or took into consideration these differences so that, in essence, similar types of patients were compared between the two settings in analyzing quality of care.

Some of the more useful process measures of quality analyzed involved the frequency with which certain types of services were provided. For example, the frequency of physician visits and the frequency of laboratory services were compared for nursing home patients and swing-bed patients. In addition, process quality scores were computed for purposes of comparing the adequacy of various types of nursing and therapy services provided to swing-bed patients and nursing home patients. Structural measures analyzed included indicators of availability of key long-term care services such as physical therapy, speech therapy, and activities programs.

To examine utilization outcomes, we collected primary data for patients in four different problem cohorts: hip fracture, confusion, incontinence, and stroke. We found that long-term care patients in swing-bed hospitals were discharged home sooner and more often than nursing home patients—even taking into consideration the differences in case mix (or risk factors) between the two patient groups. These results were obtained using a longitudinal admission sample of swing-bed patients and nursing home patients who were followed weekly for six weeks after admission. We also found that swing-bed hospital patients were hospitalized less frequently than nursing home patients by analyzing weekly data for a period of six weeks after admission and using a second sample of nursing home and swing-bed patients who were followed monthly for six months after admission.

Using a summary measure of activities of daily living (ADLs) that encompassed basic functional needs such as the ability to bathe and feed oneself, we found that swing-bed patients improved sooner and more frequently than nursing home patients, once again taking into consideration case-mix differences between the two patient types. The case-mix or risk factor–adjustment procedures also took into consideration the fact that there was a difference between swing-bed and nursing home patients in functional abilities and rehabilitation prognosis at time of admission. This result persisted for all patient cohorts pooled, and within each cohort considered separately. The findings on improved functioning also persisted for patients in the six-week longitudinal admission sample and the six-month longitudinal admission sample. Restricting analyses to Medicare patients only, for example, we found greater and more rapid improvement in functioning for swing-bed hospital patients than nursing home patients, again after adjusting for risk factors. Considering all patients (i.e., not only Medicare patients), the same results persisted in the six-week longitudinal admission sample, with swing-bed patients improving more rapidly and more frequently in terms of the summary measure of ADLs, after adjusting for differences in risk factors.

An analogous result was found for the toileting ADL (i.e., degree of patient dependence in getting to and from the bathroom or use of a bedside commode). In general, we analyzed outcomes for a number of ADLs and selected instrumental activities of daily living (IADLs; e.g., ability to use a telephone, handle one's finances), with swing-bed patients typically recovering sooner and more frequently during the first six weeks and during the first six months. In some instances, no differences were found between swing-bed and nursing home patients. For example, no differences in rates of improvement were found between swing-bed patients and nursing home patients for skin ulcers, tissue fluid swelling, and urinary tract infections. Analogously, differences were not found in the areas of cognitive, social, and environmental difficulties or dependencies—possibly due to less precise measures in these areas. When differences in patient status outcomes occurred, however, the uniform tendency was for swing-bed patients to improve sooner and more frequently than nursing home patients.

The patient status outcome results involving improvement and stabilization patterns in ADLs and IADLs reinforced those just discussed. In particular, swing-bed patients in both the six-week and six-month longitudinal admission samples generally improved or stabilized more frequently than nursing home patients, again controlling for risk factors and patient differences in initial levels of disability. One exception to this was a somewhat borderline result (in terms of statistical significance) suggesting that nursing home patients exhibited a stronger stabilization pattern than swing-bed patients in decubitus ulcers. This finding was consistent with the process quality results that implied nursing home staff provide better repositioning services than swing-bed hospital staff because of their chronic care orientation.

Several other analyses were undertaken to examine patient status outcomes, including an assessment of the percentage of time that swing-bed patients and nursing home patients spent in an improved or stabilized condition over the follow-up period (i.e., six weeks or six months, depending on the sample). The results were once again consistent with those already discussed, reinforcing the findings that swing-bed patients generally improved more frequently and more rapidly than nursing home patients in various physiologic measures of patient status, including functional measures of patient health status.

The process quality analyses revealed that physician visits occurred approximately ten times as frequently for swing-bed patients as for nursing home patients (about ten times per month versus once a month). In addition, swing-bed patients generally received more lab tests and x-rays, as well as more therapeutic and prophylactic antibiotics for urinary tract infection. Long-term care patients in swing beds generally received more fluids and more medications intravenously than nursing home patients. After case-mix adjustment, however, the differences between swing-bed patients and nursing home patients were eliminated for IV fluids and both therapeutic and prophylactic antibiotics for urinary tract infection.

Taken alone, these results on services might suggest overuse of services in swing-bed hospitals. On the other hand, taken in the context of the outcome findings, they tend to reflect a stronger therapeutic and, very likely, more aggressive approach to treating near-acute problems in swing-bed hospitals than in nursing homes. In fact, the entire profile of outcomes and process quality findings suggests that the more rehabilitation-oriented and therapeutic philosophy of care that characterizes an acute care setting carried over to near-acute patients receiving long-term care in hospital swing beds, with the result that more patients were rehabilitated in the swing-bed setting. It appears that the curative or rehabilitative philosophy that characterizes acute care is at the basis of a tendency for swing-bed hospitals to discharge long-term care patients to an independent living situation more frequently, to result in fewer rehospitalizations, and to improve patient functioning to a greater extent than was found for nursing home patients. This is beneficial from the viewpoints of enhancing of quality of life and cost containment.

Additional process quality analyses that focused on nursing services and certain therapies revealed a tendency for nursing homes to provide higher-quality chronic care services than swing-bed hospitals. This finding was consistent with the results from the swing-bed demonstration programs in the 1970s. In general, however, less emphasis was placed on the process quality results than the outcome results for the reasons discussed above.

The analyses involving structural quality measures indicated that swing-bed hospitals in the mid-1980s improved substantially relative to the demonstration hospitals of the 1970s in the extent to which they satisfied several key certification standards in the areas of physical therapy, speech therapy, occupational therapy, dental services, social services, and patient activities. By the mid-1980s, swing-bed hospitals satisfied such standards with about the same frequency as the original comparison nursing homes. In contrast to the long-term care patients discharged from swing-bed hospitals in the 1970s, nearly all long-term care patients discharged from swing-bed hospitals now have written discharge plans. In fact, of patients discharged home, significantly more swing-bed patients have written discharge plans than nursing home patients, a distinct reversal from the 1970s. (RWJF swing-bed hospitals had a higher proportion of patients discharged home with written discharge plans than other swing-bed hospitals in the mid-1980s.) Concern continues, however, that social services and patient activities may be inadequate, especially in those swing-bed hospitals where higher proportions of more traditional long-term care are provided.

Earlier data from the demonstrations in the 1970s indicated that a per capita increase in the number of Medicare SNF patients receiving care in their home community occurred as a result of the swing-bed approach. This result was replicated in the national program, with the overall finding that the availability of swing beds results in greater access to long-term care services for residents of rural communities. In terms of the present program, over 75 percent of nurses and 90 percent of physicians in swing-bed communities estimate that the swing-bed program enhanced the retention of long-term care patients in their home communities.

After obtaining the above results on quality of and access to care, we contacted a number of physicians and nurses familiar with the swing-bed program and nursing home care in swing-bed communities. Such providers, particularly physicians who were in a position to know more about patient outcomes after discharge (patients in the longitudinal samples were followed for six weeks or six months depending on the nature of the sample), generally concurred that the results were reasonable and in keeping with their assessment of swing-bed care relative to nursing home care. In all, the evidence gathered in the context of evaluating the quality of long-term care provided in hospital swing beds demonstrated that swing-bed care is of significantly higher quality than nursing home care for patients who require near-acute care. The question of whether such care is cost-effective, however, required a thorough analysis of the cost of providing swing-bed care.

CHAPTER 6

Cost of Swing-Bed Care
in the United States

This chapter presents findings on the incremental cost of swing-bed care, the relationship between incremental cost and the volume of care provided, reimbursement issues, and the cost of hospital swing-bed care to the Medicare and Medicaid programs. In view of the findings in the preceding chapter on the quality of swing-bed care, it is particularly important to examine financial issues. In doing so, it is necessary to cover a number of technical topics. For the reader who prefers not to peruse the more technical findings, the first two sections, "Cost and Cost-Effectiveness Issues" and "Reimbursement Methodology and Cost Estimation," provide an overview of the context and technical approaches. Thereafter, the chapter summary highlights the main findings and conclusions. It is possible to read only the summary for a brief overview of the results and conclusions.

COST AND COST-EFFECTIVENESS ISSUES

Incremental Cost and Reimbursement Considerations

As our need for institutional long-term care continues to increase due to our expanding elderly population, the question of how to satisfy this need most cost-effectively increases in importance. Can we avoid build-

Selected material from this chapter was published in R. Schlenker and P. Shaughnessy, "Swing-Bed Hospital Cost and Reimbursement," and is reprinted with permission from *Inquiry* 26: 508–521 (Winter 1989), © Blue Cross and Blue Shield Association. I wish to acknowledge the analytic insights, writing, and collaboration of my colleague, Robert E. Schlenker, in the financial analyses presented in this chapter.

ing an excessive number of new nursing home beds, thereby preventing a possible overbedding crisis in long-term care similar to that which occurred in the hospital field after the demand for hospital care lessened with new approaches to paying for and providing acute care? Using hospital beds to provide long-term care, if hospitals are capable of providing adequate long-term care in such beds, represents one potential way to avoid building new nursing home beds. Yet the hospital industry contends that it is more costly to operate hospital beds than nursing home beds, and that the cost of long-term care is therefore more expensive in hospital beds than in nursing home beds. This translates into higher reimbursement for long-term care provided in hospital beds than in nursing home beds.

More intense patient needs for long-term care patients would perhaps justify such a request. However, the idea that acute care is more complex to administer, the technology associated with acute care is more costly, and staffing for acute care is more complex—and should therefore translate into higher reimbursement for long-term care provided in acute care beds—is not necessarily reasonable. If hospital beds already exist to provide acute care, and the staffing and technology associated with these beds is supposedly built into reimbursement for acute care, then the marginal cost of using these beds, staff, and technology to provide long-term care should be reasonably low. One might expect such costs to parallel those of nursing homes with the same case mix. Essential, however, would be the calculation of marginal cost.

If the incremental or add-on cost of providing long-term care in acute care beds could be calculated, then reimbursement policy could be formulated so that long-term care reimbursement would cover incremental cost. The evaluation studies of the swing-bed demonstrations in the 1970s had used a methodology for estimating incremental cost. Would reapplication (and possible refinements) of this methodology confirm the prior cost estimates under the national program? Avoiding the construction of new long-term care beds by reimbursing for long-term care in acute care beds based on incremental cost might represent a long-run savings for our health care delivery system. The publicly financed Medicare and Medicaid programs could perhaps save considerably if this approach were to prove successful.

Would it be more costly to adopt the swing-bed approach, however, because of the potential double-dipping incentive mentioned in Chapters 4 and 5? That is, in addition to the likely concern that would be expressed by hospital staff that even their incremental costs are high compared with full costs for nursing homes, would we be confronted with hospitals gaming Medicare's prospective payment system by readmitting patients to acute care from long-term care provided in hospital swing beds?

Cost Effectiveness

Hospitals already have an option either to provide long-term care in existing hospital-based nursing homes or to convert hospitals beds to long-term care beds. Why not use this option instead of bothering with the swing-bed approach? The findings presented later in this chapter show there is good reason from the viewpoint of cost effectiveness to use swing beds for both acute care and long-term care. However, is there not a point at which hospitals should convert acute care beds to nursing home beds if they are constantly providing a given volume of nursing home care in those beds? The cost component of our national swing-bed program evaluation was designed to address such questions.

Hospital costs, cost to Medicare and Medicaid, the adequacy of reimbursement, the impact of swing-bed revenues on the financial positions of hospitals, and the cost of maintaining the swing-bed program relative to the alternative of building new nursing home beds were all included under the objectives of the cost component of the evaluation study. We had hoped that the aforementioned quality component of the national evaluation would yield reasonably clear results on the effectiveness of swing-bed care (something that did occur). Our plan was to combine the effectiveness findings with those from the cost component to produce a reasonably comprehensive cost-effectiveness analysis of the national swing-bed program in terms of its costs and benefits to Medicare and Medicaid, and most importantly, to patients and elderly residents of rural communities.

The cost component of the national evaluation study was also designed to shed light on the effects of the RWJF model program. Since hospital financial and administrative staff had expressed serious reservations about reimbursement and cost issues throughout the demonstration projects, these reservations had the potential to serve as a serious impediment to the national swing-bed program. The initial experiences of the RWJF model hospitals and the dissemination efforts surrounding both these experiences and information obtained from the 1970 demonstration programs would, if successful, help minimize this impediment. Thus, the extent to which hospitals would participate in the national program and, at the same time, be able to deal effectively with reimbursement-related issues, would be an indication of the success of the RWJF program.

REIMBURSEMENT METHODOLOGY AND COST ESTIMATION

Swing-Bed Reimbursement under the National Program

Medicare and Medicaid reimbursement for swing-bed hospitals is based on the incremental cost premise just discussed. The per diem reimbursement rate for swing-bed care is state specific: a given year's Medicare and Medicaid swing-bed SNF rate and the Medicaid ICF rate, if appropriate, are set at the state's average Medicaid SNF and ICF rates, respectively, for the preceding year. Some variations exist in terms of Medicaid rate setting in this regard, and, as mentioned, some state Medicaid programs do not participate at all in the swing-bed program. The key assumption in establishing swing-bed reimbursement rates in this manner is that the preceding year's Medicaid nursing home rates adequately cover incremental costs.

With the implementation of Medicare's prospective payment system (PPS), the initial approach to swing-bed reimbursement under the national program became more financially attractive to hospitals. The original approach included a carve-out method (Pennell 1982) that reduced reimbursable costs for acute care by the estimated swing-bed long-term care revenues received from all payers. This was akin to the formula used in the Iowa Swing-Bed Project (ISBP) in the 1970s. Under PPS, the carve-out became relatively inconsequential in dollar terms since it was only continued for capital and medical education reimbursement. Since routine operating cost reimbursement for acute care was no longer reduced, swing-bed care became financially more attractive to hospitals. Despite this change, hospital administrators surveyed during the national evaluation continued to indicate that reimbursement for swing-bed care was inadequate (Shaughnessy, Schlenker, et al. 1985). The changed reimbursement environment and differing opinions regarding the adequacy of swing-bed reimbursement highlighted the importance of estimating the cost of swing-bed routine care, and of estimating the relationship of cost to revenues received.

Swing-bed ancillary service cost and reimbursement are also important. Ancillary services include physical therapy, laboratory services, medical supplies, and other such services. This is primarily a Medicare issue, since Medicare is the major purchaser of ancillary services for swing-bed and many other SNF patients over age 65. Ancillary service reimbursement for swing-bed care is based on the proportion of the hospital's ancillary costs that are attributable to swing-bed patients, determined using a pre-PPS method. Since ancillary services for Medicare acute patients are now part of the diagnosis-related group payment, a financial incentive, as discussed earlier, exists to shift patients from acute to swing-bed status quickly, and to maximize the provision of ancillary services when the patient is receiving swing-bed long-term care. As with routine care, these PPS-induced incentives stimulated heightened interest in the analysis of swing-bed ancillary costs and reimbursement in the evaluation study.

Cost Data and Estimation Procedures

Data and Hospitals. The primary data set used for the cost and reimbursement analyses involved Medicare cost reports and related information for a sample of 150 hospitals (75 swing-bed and 75 comparison non-swing-bed hospitals) located in 27 states. Data were used for fiscal years 1982 and 1984. The comparison hospitals were eligible but not participating in the swing-bed program and were located predominantly in the same states as the sample swing-bed hospitals. Swing-bed hospitals in the sample were generally representative of all swing-bed hospitals in 1984. Analyses were conducted comparing sample swing-bed hospitals with other swing-bed hospitals at that time, using available American Hospital Association data on characteristics such as size, ownership, and occupancy rates. Similar analyses were carried out for the swing-bed and comparison hospitals in 1982. The swing-bed and comparison hospitals were similar in terms of most characteristics, particularly their cost structures, prior to the start of the swing-bed program in 1982.

Of the 75 swing-bed hospitals, 69 reported swing-bed utilization in 1984, with swing-bed days ranging from 42 to 4,285, averaging 1,145 days. The incremental cost estimates were derived using this subsample of 69 hospitals, which included 22 RWJF grantee hospitals.

Incremental Cost Estimation. When a swing-bed hospital files its Medicare cost report, the cost of swing-bed routine care is included with all other routine costs. In the financial component of the national swing-bed evaluation, it was therefore necessary to develop estimation methods to separate the incremental cost of providing swing-bed care from all other routine costs. The demonstration project evaluation (Shaughnessy et al. 1980a, 1980b) had developed an accounting estimation methodology that allocated the costs of selected overhead cost centers to routine care, and then apportioned the resulting costs to swing-bed care using the ratio of swing-bed to total inpatient days. A variant of this approach was used in the national evaluation, expanding the methodology to include new overhead cost centers as well as new allocation and apportionment techniques.

The major accounting methods used are summarized in Table 6.1. Regression techniques were also applied using both the swing-bed and

Table 6.1   Allocation and Apportionment Methods Used to Estimate
Swing-Bed Incremental Routine Cost

Overhead Cost Centers Allocated to the Routine Cost Center	Allocation Basis	Apportionment Method and Cost Centers Included		
		Method 1	Method 2	Method 3
Administrative and general	Cost net of admin. cost		DD1	DD2
Maintenance and repairs	Revenue-producing square feet	DD1	DD1	DD2
Operation of plant	Revenue-producing square feet	DD1	DD1	DD2
Laundry and linen	Pounds of laundry	DD1	DD1	DD1-2
Housekeeping	Revenue-producing square feet	DD1	DD1	DD1-2
Dietary	Meals	DD1	DD1	DD1-2
Nursing administration	Nursing time		DD1	DD2
Central services and supply	Costed supply requisitions			DD2
Medical records	Revenue-producing net cost		DD1	DD2
Social services	Revenue-producing net cost		DD1	DD2
Direct routine cost		DD1	DD1	DD2

Notes: Method used to attribute (apportion) costs to swing-bed care: DD1 = the swing-bed to total routine days ratio; DD2 = the square of the swing-bed to total routine days ratio; DD1-2 = the DD1 ratio for nonlabor and the DD2 ratio for labor in these cost centers. Methods 1 and 2 include only nonlabor costs. Method 3 includes both nonlabor and labor costs.

Source: Reprinted with permission from *Inquiry* 26: 508–521 (Winter 1989), © Blue Cross and Blue Shield Association.

comparison hospital samples to estimate and compare cost functions for routine care. In regressions involving the swing-bed hospital sample, variables were included to separate the effects of swing-bed care from acute care. In the discussion of findings presented in the next section, emphasis is placed on the results from the accounting methods in Table 6.1; regression methods were used primarily to confirm and interpret the accounting method findings. The resulting estimates are based on combining the skilled and intermediate levels of care, but pertain primarily to skilled care since, as noted in earlier chapters, most swing-bed patients received skilled care.

Methods 1 and 2 assumed that only nonlabor costs vary with swing-bed care. Such costs were attributed (apportioned) to swing-bed care by assuming that acute and swing-bed patients incur the same costs in the cost centers shown in Table 6.1 (i.e., using a days-to-days apportionment methodology). A major difference between the two methods is that method 2 added four additional overhead cost centers, the most expensive of which was the administrative and general cost center. The added costs of method 2 were judged to be reasonable components of swing-bed incremental costs.

Method 3 incorporated labor costs, but generally apportioned costs to swing-bed care in a manner different from the first two methods. The basic concept underlying method 3 is that costs are apportioned to swing-bed care in the same proportion as the squared ratio of swing-bed to total inpatient days. Thus, if swing-bed days represented 30 percent of total days, then $.30 \times .30 = .09$, or 9 percent of costs were attributed to swing-bed care. The approach taken in method 3 therefore recognized labor costs as potentially influencing incremental costs, but in keeping with our time study done during the Utah demonstration program, took into consideration the lesser amounts of staff time required by swing-bed patients (relative to acute care patients). This apportionment method resulted in low swing-bed costs per day for hospitals with low swing-bed volume and higher costs per day for higher volume hospitals. This was in keeping with the observed phenomenon that per unit incremental cost was quite low when negligible amounts of swing-bed care were provided, but higher when more days of swing-bed care (relative to acute care) were provided. Exceptions to this apportionment approach in method 3 were made for the nonlabor costs in laundry, housekeeping, and dietary cost centers. The nonlabor costs in these categories were assumed to be the same for swing-bed and acute care patients and were therefore apportioned using the days-to-days ratio.

The results from apportionment method 3 were consistent with anecdotal evidence and findings from other investigations. For example, surveys of swing-bed hospital administrators and case studies were undertaken at individual swing-bed hospitals to obtain additional information on this topic. These sources supported the assumption that the per day nonlabor costs in the dietary, laundry and linen, and housekeeping cost centers were usually the same for swing-bed and acute care patients. Other nonlabor costs were estimated by most respondents to be considerably lower for swing-bed than for acute care patients. Labor costs, particularly for nursing staff, were estimated to be low for small amounts of swing-bed care, confirming the results of the more formal time study conducted as part of the Utah evaluation during the 1970s. In view of the need for 24-hour nursing coverage by acute care hospitals, nursing staff coverage tended to be more than adequate for swing beds at low acute census levels. The anecdotal evidence tended to demonstrate that small numbers of swing-bed patients could therefore usually be accommodated without increasing nursing staff costs. As swing-bed volume increased to moderate levels, the major nursing staff increase typically was in the aide category, which tended not to increase costs greatly.

Although hospital staff could not estimate precisely the labor and nonlabor increases required for high volumes of swing-bed care, generally due to lack of experience with high volumes of swing-bed care, most indicated that such added resources would be increasingly costly as excess capacity (in both labor and nonlabor) was used up. Also, regression estimates suggested that swing-bed cost per day was likely to increase as volume increased. Several ways were considered and tested to capture this phenomenon of marginal cost, especially labor cost, increasing as a function of the proportion of inpatient care provided to swing-bed patients. The square of the days-to-days ratio, for the indicated cost centers, was selected since it reflected how costs were being incurred—conceptually as well as empirically. The overall conclusion based on these varied sources of information was that a reasonable apportionment method, such as method 3, should include labor costs, but higher costs per day should be apportioned to swing-bed care as swing-bed volume increased. As a corollary to developing the approach for method 3, we concluded that for some of the cost centers (those other than laundry, dietary, and housekeeping), we were probably generous in methods 1 and 2 when applying the days-to-days (i.e., unsquared) apportionment method. However, this was offset by not including labor costs when using these methods.

COST AND REIMBURSEMENT FINDINGS

Incremental Routine Cost and Reimbursement

The incremental routine cost estimates derived from the three accounting methods are presented in Table 6.2. The average incremental cost estimates ranged from $22.11 to $34.05 per day. While the average for method 3 was close to that for method 2, it is important to recall that method 3 used additional cost centers and apportioned costs to swing-bed care under the assumption that certain types of costs increase more rapidly as the volume (number of days) of swing-bed care increases. Because the average values for these three methods were influenced by high estimated values for a few hospitals, medians are also presented in Table 6.2. The medians were lower than the means for all three methods,

Table 6.2   Swing-Bed Incremental Routine Cost and Revenue per Day
for 69 Swing-Bed Hospitals, 1984

	Method 1	Method 2	Method 3
Estimated routine cost per day			
Mean	$22.11	$32.69	$34.05
Median	18.35	27.55	32.30
Routine revenue per day*	44.10	44.10	44.10
Revenue minus estimated cost†	21.99	11.41	10.05
Revenue minus cost, adjusted for the capital and medical education carve-out‡	20.30	9.72	8.36

*This is the average routine revenue per day estimated for each hospital in the swing-bed adjustment process associated with the Medicare cost report. This estimate assumes that all swing-bed days (regardless of payer) are paid at the statewide average Medicaid rates for the prior calendar year by level of care (skilled and intermediate). One hospital had missing data for this variable. That case was assumed to have the average revenue value derived for the remaining 68 cases.

†These values were calculated as the average routine revenue amount for all hospitals minus the average estimated routine cost for all hospitals.

‡Medicare reimbursement for acute capital and medical education costs deducts (carves out) a portion of such costs as attributable to swing-bed care. The proportion of the carved-out amount that represents a reduction in revenue to a swing-bed hospital is equal to the ratio of Medicare to total acute care days in the facility. The average reduction for the 69 swing-bed hospitals was $1.69 per swing-bed day.

Source: Reprinted with permission from *Inquiry* 26: 508–521 (Winter 1989), © Blue Cross and Blue Shield Association.

indicating that the averages overstate slightly the incremental costs actually incurred by most hospitals. In fact, most hospitals had estimated incremental costs of less than $40 per swing-bed day (90 percent were less $40 for method 1, 77 percent for method 2, and 70 percent for method 3). To allow for some degree of imprecision involved in any estimation method and the possibility that the methods did not fully capture the added costs resulting from the provision of swing-bed care, mean values are used in the subsequent discussion, with emphasis on the estimates derived using methods 2 and 3.

The incremental cost estimates for routine care presented in Table 6.2 were compared with estimates of revenues received by swing-bed hospitals to assess whether swing-bed revenues covered the incremental costs of swing-bed care. Although reliable data on swing-bed revenues from all payers were not available from the cost reports, estimates were derived from the swing-bed adjustment utilized in the Medicare carve-out procedure. That procedure applies the average state Medicaid rates for the prior year by level of care to all swing-bed patients (the revenue estimates were developed as weighted averages incorporating the rates for both levels of care). Since Medicare and most Medicaid programs reimburse using these rates, the resulting revenue estimates were fairly accurate for Medicare and Medicaid. For other payers and private-pay patients, these rates were reasonable estimates according to information received from swing-bed providers and other sources. The resulting swing-bed revenues ranged from $29.34 to $107.00, averaging $44.10 per day. The wide variation among hospitals in revenue per day reflects the wide variation in average Medicaid rates across the country.

Average revenues were found to exceed average cost by $10 to $22 per day, depending on the incremental cost estimation method. For methods 2 and 3, which were considered to yield the more realistic estimates, revenues exceeded costs by average per diem amounts of $11.41 and $10.05, respectively. Although the averages indicated overall financial gains for swing-bed hospitals, several hospitals had costs greater than revenues. The estimated numbers of hospitals with such losses were 2, 11, and 22 for methods 1, 2, and 3, respectively. For method 3, the method yielding the most hospitals with financial losses, the hospitals incurring such losses generally tended to provide higher volumes of swing-bed care. This is consistent with the premise (built into the estimation methodology) that incremental cost increases with volume.

The last row in Table 6.2 adjusts the financial gain (or loss) to incorporate the capital and medical education carve-out applied by Medicare. The procedure, described in the notes to the table, reduced Medicare acute care reimbursement. The reduction depends on the hospital's total capital costs, the ratio of estimated swing-bed to total routine costs, and the proportion of acute care days that are Medicare days. With this adjustment, the average financial gains dropped to $9.72 and $8.36 for methods 2 and 3, respectively. The number of hospitals with losses increased slightly, to 4, 16, and 23 under methods 1, 2, and 3, respectively. Thus, these findings suggest that in 1984 most swing-bed hospitals received routine care revenues that exceeded the incremental cost of routine care, even with the adjustment for the capital and medical education carve-out. Such gains did not have a major impact on the financial status of most hospitals. Even with the inclusion of swing-bed ancillary revenues (discussed later in this chapter), swing-bed revenues typically represented less than 5 percent of total 1984 patient revenues for the average hospital. As we will see, the losses sustained by a somewhat significant minority of hospitals, depending on the incremental cost estimation used, relate to the volume of swing-bed care provided; these losses were partially offset by gains in ancillary care revenues for several hospitals.

Incremental Routine Cost and Volume

The association of swing-bed cost and volume is important to both hospitals and policymakers. When swing-bed care reaches a certain volume (in patient days), that portion of a swing-bed hospital used to provide such care (be it physically distinct or simply a fraction of total resources available) may be functioning almost as a nursing home in terms of resources consumed and its overall cost structure. Under such circumstances, physically converting acute care beds to long-term care beds, thereby transforming a portion of the hospital into a certified distinct-part hospital-based nursing home, may be advisable.

Since most sample hospitals provided relatively small amounts of swing-bed care in 1984, the association between volume and cost was difficult to determine. Method 3 had the most reasonable pattern of results (and underlying assumptions) for analyzing the relationship between incremental cost and volume. Consequently, the following inferences about the association of swing-bed incremental cost with volume are based on the method 3 approach. Table 6.3 presents regression-based estimates of average and marginal swing-bed incremental costs per day for different volumes of swing-bed care. The equations relating average and marginal costs to swing-bed volume are shown in the footnotes to the table. The average cost column shows the mean incremental

Table 6.3 Swing-Bed Volume and Cost: Illustrative Average and Marginal Swing-Bed Incremental Routine Cost per Day for 69 Swing-Bed Hospitals, 1984

Swing-Bed Days	Average Incremental Cost*	Marginal Incremental Cost†
500	$26.69	$32.19
1,000	32.19	43.19
1,500	37.69	54.19
2,000	43.19	65.19
3,000	54.19	87.19

*These estimates are based on the estimated regression equation: SBAC = 21.186 + .011(SBD), where SBAC = estimated method 3 average incremental routine cost per day, the constant term is actually several facility characteristics estimated at mean values, and SBD = swing-bed days. The R^2 for this equation was .461.

†Using the equation in the preceding footnote for the average cost per swing-bed day, the marginal cost of each added swing-bed day can be derived as SBMC = 21.186 + .022(SBD). See Schlenker and Shaughnessy (1989) for this derivation.

Source: Reprinted with permission from *Inquiry* 26: 508–521 (Winter 1989), © Blue Cross and Blue Shield Association.

cost per day of all swing-bed days at each respective volume. The marginal cost column of the table indicates the added cost for each additional swing-bed day of care at different volumes. For instance, based on these equations, a hospital providing 1,000 days of swing-bed care had an average 1984 cost of $32.19 and a marginal cost (for an additional swing-bed day beyond 1,000) of $43.19.

These estimated relationships were used to examine the relationship between financial gain (or loss) and volume. Break-even volumes were calculated for marginal and average costs at different payment rate amounts. Using marginal cost for instance, at the mean 1984 payment amount of about $45 per day, the average hospital was estimated to incur a per day loss for each additional swing-bed day beyond 1,082. Overall, however, the provision of swing-bed care would still have resulted in a net financial gain to such hospitals, until the point at which the average incremental cost (not the marginal cost) exceeded the payment rate—about 2,165 days. Although these estimates must be considered approximations, they suggest that about 1,000 swing-bed days (which was the average number of swing-bed days per hospital in 1985, noted in Chapter 4) is close to the estimated marginal cost break-even volume. More importantly, however, most hospitals would very likely experience a net financial gain for volumes up to approximately 2,000 days, the average cost break-even volume.

Clearly, swing-bed hospital staff should not necessarily base decisions solely on financial factors, and most do not make such precise calculations as illustrated here. Nevertheless, these findings suggest that unless hospitals can prevent marginal costs from increasing with volume, they will benefit financially from the provision of swing-bed care mainly at low volumes. If a hospital provides sufficiently high volumes of swing-bed care (e.g., beyond 2,000–2,500 days of such care, depending on its state-specific reimbursement rate), it may be advisable to establish a distinct-part unit, taking into consideration the extent to which this would compromise the acute care bed supply in the hospital.

Swing-Bed Costs Relative to SNF Costs

Table 6.4 contains estimates of the cost to Medicare of SNF care in swing-bed hospitals compared with rural SNF units (both freestanding and hospital based) in 1984. The SNF swing-bed routine operating cost payment rates were averaged for all states. A weighted average was derived using the number of Medicare swing-bed patient days for each state from the cost report sample. The mean capital and medical education carve-out deduction per Medicare swing-bed day was subtracted (from both the

Table 6.4   Medicare per Diem SNF Routine Care Reimbursement for Rural Swing-Bed, Freestanding, and Hospital-Based Units, 1984

	Swing-Bed	Freestanding	Hospital-Based
Average state rates	$43.52	$51.51*	$79.60*
Weighted sample average rates†	43.04	49.77	68.76

Freestanding (%)	Hospital-Based (%)	Swing-Bed Rate	Alternative Rate	Medicare Savings per Day of Swing-Bed Care‡
100	0	$43.04	$49.77	$ 6.73
50	50	43.04	59.27	16.23
0	100	43.04	68.76	25.72

Notes: Swing-bed reimbursement rates for 1984 (SNF level) were obtained from HCFA regional offices and individual state Medicaid programs. These rates were averaged across states and then reduced by the average Medicare acute capital and medical education reimbursement deduction per Medicare swing-bed day. The reduction was noted in Table 6.2 to average $1.69 per all-payer swing-bed day. For this sample, considering Medicare only, that amount converts to $4.87 per Medicare swing-bed day, which is the appropriate amount to use in comparing Medicare reimbursement in alternative settings.

*The average operating costs for rural freestanding and hospital-based Medicare SNFs were estimated using data from the Medicare cost limit derivations for hospital-based SNFs for 1982–84 and for freestanding and hospital-based SNFs for 1986, both published in the *Federal Register*, Vol. 51, No. 62, April 1, 1986, pp. 11234–11264. For each set of limits, rural mean cost values were derived, inflated or deflated to the fiscal period 10/1/83–9/30/84, adjusted by the appropriate state rural wage index for labor cost components, and averaged across states. Capital-related costs, including return on equity (ROE), were estimated from the calculations underlying the 1986 Medicare SNF prospective payment rates for rural areas (see *Medicare Provider Reimbursement Manual*, Part I, Transmittal No. 337, HCFA-Pub. 15-1, August 1986). The capital-related cost data were assumed to approximate reasonably well the capital-related amounts of SNFs in 1984. The capital cost data were derived for each state, averaged across states, then adjusted to mean values. Since the variation across states was minimal, the resulting state rural average of $4.70 per patient day was used for this table. The Medicare return on equity rural average for 1984 was estimated as $1.16 per day. Since most freestanding SNFs are proprietary and most hospital-based SNFs are not, the $1.16 ROE was included in the capital-related estimate for freestanding SNFs and excluded for hospital-based units.

†The weighted rates were calculated using the number of Medicare swing-bed days reported by the 64 of the 69 swing-bed hospitals (in cost report sample) with Medicare swing-bed days in fiscal year 1984. For the swing-bed, freestanding, and hospital-based operating cost reimbursement components, each state rate was weighted by the number of Medicare swing-bed days in the sample facilities for that state. The capital components were then incorporated in the same manner as was done for the average state rates.

‡This calculation uses the weighted sample average rates and assumes that patients not receiving swing-bed care would receive the same number of days of Medicare SNF care in either freestanding or hospital-based rural facilities, with Medicare reimbursement at the average Medicare rural SNF cost. Alternative distributions of those SNF days between freestanding and hospital-based units are presented.

Source: Reprinted with permission from *Inquiry* 26: 508–521 (Winter 1989), © Blue Cross and Blue Shield Association.

state and weighted-average rates) to derive rates that would be comparable to the alternative SNF rates that also include a capital component.

HCFA data on the Medicare routine operating cost limits in rural areas for freestanding and hospital-based SNFs were used to obtain estimates of average routine operating costs for the 1983–1984 fiscal period covered by the sample Medicare cost reports. Mean values were derived for each state to approximate alternative Medicare SNF reimbursement amounts. The results were averaged in the same two ways as the swing-bed rates. Capital reimbursement estimates (including a return on equity for proprietary facilities) were added to the estimated average operating costs.

The weighted rates were used to estimate the differences between the swing-bed payment per day and the likely alternative for swing-bed patients. In view of the near-acute case mix for swing-bed patients, it was assumed that many such patients would typically need care in hospital-based rather than freestanding facilities. If the alternative was hospital-based SNF care for all Medicare swing-bed patients, then the estimated Medicare savings from the swing-bed program per day in 1984 would have been $25.72. If the swing-bed patients had been equally divided between freestanding and hospital-based rural Medicare SNF facilities, then the Medicare savings would have been $16.23 per day. Even if all swing-bed patients had been placed in freestanding SNFs, a highly unlikely event, Medicare would have still saved $6.73 per Medicare swing-bed day. These comparisons therefore suggest that swing-bed care resulted in reduced cost to Medicare under the assumption that Medicare swing-bed SNF patients would have been SNF patients in a nursing home had they not received SNF care in swing beds. Using the equal split between hospital-based and freestanding units as a reasonable possibility, the amount of the savings to Medicare would have been about $16 per Medicare swing-bed day in 1984.

After 1984, however, the Medicare savings for swing-bed patients who would have otherwise been in hospital-based facilities may have been lower (before adjusting for inflation) than in 1984 because the reimbursement limits for hospital-based SNFs were lowered. Nonetheless, the above approach may underestimate the Medicare savings for two reasons. First, a substantial proportion of swing-bed patients might have alternatively received care in urban SNF facilities, at correspondingly higher reimbursement rates. The earlier-cited results from the community retention analyses done as part of the evaluation indicated that a reasonably large number of patients who would have received SNF care in more distant urban areas now receive such care in swing beds in rural communities. Second, the preceding estimates include average capital costs for nursing home care. In the absence of the swing-bed program, however, nursing home construction or expansion may have increased, with correspondingly higher capital costs. For example, Finkler (1987) estimated the capital costs of new nursing home construction at around $10.90 per patient day during this period. This amount would represent an increase of $6.20 per patient day over the capital estimates in the notes to Table 6.4.

Ancillary Care Revenues: Attractive for Swing-Bed Hospitals

Medicare swing-bed ancillary cost and charge information was available in the Medicare cost reports. Originally, nineteen ancillary cost centers were examined. Nine of these combined to add average Medicare ancillary service reimbursement amounts of less than 10 cents per Medicare swing-bed day. Several of the remaining ten services had highly skewed distributions in terms of reimbursement for each cost center. As a result, we employed the criterion that at least ten hospitals must have ancillary reimbursement amounts per Medicare swing-bed day of greater than 1 cent. This removed three additional ancillary services of intravenous therapy, occupational therapy, and speech therapy. Electrocardiology was eliminated because relatively few hospitals reported swing-bed utilization for this service and the average reimbursement was only 7.4 cents per swing-bed day. Listed in Table 6.5 are the six remaining services that constituted the major swing-bed ancillary services reimbursed by Medicare.

Although overhead costs were allocated to the ancillary departments, they represented smaller proportions of ancillary service costs than was the case for routine care. Also, for five of the six ancillary services, charges for Medicare swing-bed patients represented less than 5 percent of total charges for that service. The exception was physical therapy, for which Medicare swing-bed charges averaged 12.6 percent of total physical therapy charges in the typical swing-bed hospital. Consequently, it was clear that the incremental costs of ancillary services for swing-bed patients would be fairly small relative to acute care costs.

Estimates of the average incremental Medicare swing-bed ancillary costs are presented in Table 6.5. These estimates are based on three accounting methods analogous to those used for routine care. The three methods are explained in the footnotes to Table 6.5. Since hospitals characterized by low volumes of Medicare swing-bed care tended to have aberrant per day reimbursement amounts for ancillary services, we excluded hospitals with less than one month (i.e., 31 days) of swing-bed care. The results therefore pertain to 58 swing-bed hospitals.

The range in means for incremental ancillary cost across the three methods was between $15 and $21 per Medicare swing-bed day. This

Table 6.5   Medicare Swing-Bed Incremental Ancillary Cost and Reimbursement per Day for 58 Swing-Bed Hospitals, 1984

Ancillary Cost Center	Mean Dollar Values per Medicare Swing-Bed Day		
	Method 1	Method 2	Method 3
Radiology	$ .48	$ .58	$ .59
Laboratory	1.90	2.35	2.39
Respiratory therapy	1.95	2.32	2.45
Physical therapy	4.69	5.70	6.65
Medical supplies	2.40	2.78	3.02
Drugs	4.42	5.12	5.70
Total	$15.84	$18.85	$20.80
Medicare ancillary reimbursement per day	$31.55	$31.55	$31.55
Reimbursement minus estimated cost	$15.71	$12.70	$10.75

Notes: Method 1 is analogous to method 1 for routine care. It allocates costs from the same overhead cost centers as routine method 1, but apportions to swing-bed care on a charges-to-charges (rather than a days-to-days) basis. (That is, the ratio of Medicare swing-bed charges to total ancillary charges, by cost center, is used to attribute the costs of a particular ancillary cost center to Medicare swing-bed patients.) Only nonlabor costs are included.

Method 2 is analogous to method 2 for routine care, including the same overhead cost centers as routine method 2, but using the charges-to-charges apportionment method. Method 2 also includes only nonlabor costs.

Method 3 is similar to method 3 for routine care. It includes all routine method 3 overhead cost centers, plus the pharmacy cost center (which is entirely allocated to the drugs ancillary cost center). The apportionment to swing-bed care includes both nonlabor and labor. Nonlabor is apportioned on a charges-to-charges basis, while labor is apportioned using the square of the charges-to-charges ratio.

Source: Reprinted with permission from *Inquiry* 26: 508–521 (Winter 1989), © Blue Cross and Blue Shield Association.

range of estimates using the three methods is narrower than for routine care due to the diminished importance of overhead costs with respect to ancillary services. Further, unlike routine care costs, the estimates varied little as a function of swing-bed volume, because the fixed-cost component of ancillary service cost is typically much lower proportionately than the fixed cost of routine care. Since variable cost therefore accounts for a greater proportion of total cost for ancillary services, this tends to make marginal cost less sensitive to volume (within reasonable volume ranges).

Table 6.5 also compares the Medicare reimbursement amounts per day to the estimated incremental costs. The average net gain from ancillary services ranged from $10.75 for method 3 to $15.71 for method 1. Again, the estimates from methods 2 and 3 were taken as the more appropriate estimates of costs (i.e., more likely to include all costs relevant to swing-bed care). For these methods, the average net gain was roughly between $10 and $13. Thus, we concluded that ancillary service reimbursement adequately covered the incremental costs of such services for most sample hospitals in 1984. Further, given the ratio of ancillary reimbursement per day to the estimated per day incremental cost for ancillary care, it is apparent that the methodology used for ancillary reimbursement is more advantageous to hospitals than the approach to routine care reimbursement.

No Evidence of Gaming: Swing Beds are Cost-Effective

As stated earlier, under PPS swing-bed hospitals could possibly game the combined acute–swing-bed reimbursement system in two ways. First, the provision of ancillary services could be minimized during an acute stay, still enabling the hospital to receive the full DRG payment for that stay. Thereafter, the patient could be transferred to long-term care in a hospital swing bed, at which point, ancillary services could possibly be overprovided, but reimbursed according to the volume of services provided. Second, hospitals could discharge a patient from acute care to swing-bed care and then back to acute care under another DRG. This would allow the hospital to receive two separate DRG payments and a per day payment between the two acute stays for long-term care provided in swing beds. Both of these incentives to double-dip into the Medicare reimbursement system were analyzed empirically.

The patient-level findings presented earlier indicated a higher use of selected ancillary services (e.g., x-ray and lab services) by swing-bed patients than by nursing home patients. Selected differences persisted after adjusting for case mix, which could reflect either higher-quality care or overprovision of services by swing-bed hospitals. We established earlier that swing-bed patients with near-acute care needs received higher-quality care on the basis of patient outcomes, thereby suggesting that such service provision was probably warranted.

Cost report data could not be used to compare the cost of ancillary services by swing-bed patients relative to nursing home patients, since many such services for SNF patients are provided outside the facility and reimbursed separately (i.e., not as part of the SNF's cost report). However, for the study sample of swing-bed hospitals, it was possible to compare the amounts reimbursed for swing-bed ancillary services with the amounts that would have been reimbursed for the same services to acute care patients prior to PPS. These amounts represent what would have been reimbursed for Medicare acute patients under the pre-PPS cost reimbursement methodology. The results of these comparisons are presented in Table 6.6. It is evident that the total ancillary cost per day for the six most costly ancillary services provided to swing-bed patients were more than three times greater for acute care patients than for swing-bed patients. Considerably higher cost per day (due to higher use) by acute care patients was evident for five of the six individual services. The exception was physical therapy, which was more heavily utilized by swing-bed patients. This is reasonable in view of the importance of physical therapy for rehabilitation of near-acute long-term care patients.

The utilization outcome results presented earlier demonstrated that swing-bed patients tend to be rehospitalized less frequently than nursing home patients. Combined with the enhanced patient status outcomes and the increased proportion of swing-bed patients discharged home, this would not only imply potentially higher-quality care, but possibly a cost savings to the Medicare program through reduced utilization of Medicare-covered services after a swing-bed patient's initial acute care stay. This topic subsumes both the potential for increased ancillary cost to Medicare and a possible increase in total cost by virtue of re-hospitalization. To further investigate this issue, we analyzed Medicare claims data for 31,098 patients discharged from swing-bed or comparison hospitals in 1985. The hospitals used were those that were studied in the cost analyses presented earlier. This analysis examined the

Table 6.6 Medicare Acute and Swing-Bed Costs per Day for the Six Major Swing-Bed Ancillary Services for 58 Swing-Bed Hospitals, 1984

Ancillary Cost Center	Acute Costs	Swing-Bed Costs
Radiology	$ 11.56	$ 1.01
Laboratory	33.54	4.08
Respiratory therapy	15.02	3.94
Physical therapy	3.46	11.06
Medical supplies	17.58	4.84
Drugs	22.19	6.62
Total	$103.35	$31.55

Notes: Acute costs are Medicare Part A inpatient acute costs for each ancillary cost center, as determined in the Medicare cost reports, after allocation and apportionment. They are no longer separately reimbursed for PPS hospitals, but are covered under the DRG payment. Nevertheless, the cost estimates are useful here for comparative purposes.

Swing-bed costs are Medicare swing-bed ancillary costs, as determined in the Medicare cost reports, after allocation and apportionment (i.e., they are not the incremental cost estimates reported earlier, but the amounts actually reimbursed).

Source: Reprinted with permission from Inquiry 26: 508–521 (Winter 1989), © Blue Cross and Blue Shield Association.

total cost to Medicare for patients discharged from swing-bed hospitals relative to non-swing-bed hospitals. The results are summarized in Table 6.7. The analysis was conducted as part of the augmentation to the national evaluation designed to examine the combined effects of PPS and the swing-bed approach.

For the 31,098 patients, subsequent utilization and costs for Medicare services were compared for patients discharged from swing-bed hospitals relative to patients discharged from non-swing-bed hospitals in rural communities. Data covered Medicare costs and utilization for acute care (first admission and subsequent admissions), swing-bed care, other SNF care, home health care, and physician/outpatient care. The sum of the costs for all such services comprised the total Medicare patient care costs analyzed. Although swing-bed and other SNF care are both Medicare-skilled nursing care, they are treated separately in this analysis owing to the focus on swing-bed care as distinct from SNF care provided in nursing homes. Four time periods were analyzed, beginning with the date of discharge from the first acute care admission in 1985 and covering, respectively, the subsequent three months, six months, nine months, and the remainder of 1985.

The findings in terms of Medicare utilization and cost were similar for all four time periods. Consequently, the results for all of 1985 (the largest sample of patients) are presented in Table 6.7. The average costs (i.e., Medicare reimbursement) per patient associated with the initial acute admission in 1985 were similar for the two hospital types, although slightly lower for swing-bed hospitals. This small difference in cost per patient did not appear to reflect case-mix differences since the average length of stay and DRG rates were not significantly different for patients of the two hospital types. Further, the average dates of discharge were the same for patients discharged from swing-bed hospitals and those discharged from non-swing-bed hospitals, thereby precluding the possibility that higher reimbursement rates might have been in effect for one group than for the other.

The findings cited in Chapter 5 using primary data showed swing-bed patients were rehospitalized less than nursing home patients after risk factor adjustment. This is also reflected to some extent by Table 6.7: the number of subsequent hospital admissions was lower for patients whose initial discharge had been from a swing-bed hospital rather than from a non-swing-bed hospital. The per case cost for subsequent acute care was $62 lower for patients admitted to swing-bed hospitals than for non-swing-bed hospital patients.

As is evident from Table 6.7, acute care patients discharged from swing-bed hospitals tended to receive more swing-bed SNF care, less SNF care in other nursing homes, and less home health care than pa-

Table 6.7   Medicare Utilization and Reimbursement (Cost) for 31,098
Patients Discharged from Swing-Bed or Comparison
Hospitals in 1985

	Means (per Discharge)	
	Swing-Bed Hospital Patients (N = 17,534)	Comparison Hospital Patients (N = 13,564)
Initial acute care admission		
Cost per patient in sample	$ 1,747	$ 1,777
Subsequent acute care		
Percent hospitalized in 1985	59%	66%
Cost per patient in sample	$ 1,533	$ 1,595
Swing-bed SNF care		
Percent receiving swing-bed care in 1985	9%	0%*
Cost per patient in sample	$ 74.49	$ .53
Other SNF care		
Percent receiving other SNF care in 1985	3%	4%
Cost per patient in sample	$ 22.69	$ 37.34
Home health care		
Number of 1985 visits per sample patient	2.71	3.16
Cost per patient in sample	$112.34	$145.16
Total long-term care†		
Cost per patient in sample	$209.52	$183.02
Physician/outpatient care		
Part A cost per patient in sample	$136.57	$131.46
Part B cost per patient in sample	$451.34	$509.21
Cost per sample patient after initial discharge	$ 2,331	$ 2,419
Total cost per sample patient	$ 4,078	$ 4,195

Notes: The mean difference between the swing-bed and non–swing-bed patient groups
for Part A physician costs was insignificant. Differences for subsequent acute care costs
and total cost after initial discharge were significant at $p < .10$. All other differences were
significant at $p < .05$.

*This mean was less than 1%.

†Total long-term care is defined to include Medicare swing-bed, other SNF, and home
health care. It is noteworthy, however, that the higher Medicare Part B cost for comparison
hospital patients is partially attributable to Part B costs of services that were provided in
conjunction with long-term care stays in nursing home (SNFs) or while under the care of
certified home health agencies.

tients discharged from non-swing-bed hospitals. In all, the cost of Part A Medicare SNF care received after the initial hospitalization for such patients was higher for patients discharged from swing-bed hospitals, owing to the provision of more SNF care in swing beds (i.e., approximately $70 greater per patient). However, as indicated in the notes to Table 6.7, the lower Part B costs for physician/outpatient care received by patients discharged from swing-bed hospitals pertain partly to outpatient services, some of which were provided as part of the Medicare SNF stay.

Total physician and outpatient reimbursement tended to be lower for patients discharged from swing-bed hospitals. This was due to lower subsequent physician and outpatient reimbursement after discharge from acute care. Part A reimbursement was slightly higher, but insignificantly so, while Part B reimbursement was approximately $58 lower per patient.

In all, Medicare costs were less for patients discharged from swing-bed hospitals than from non-swing-bed hospitals. The Medicare savings was accounted for by virtue of a substitution of swing-bed care for both subsequent acute care and physician/outpatient care, in keeping with the findings on quality of care discussed previously. Namely, by virtue of improved rehabilitation and discharge home as a result of better rehabilitation by swing-bed hospitals, fewer hospital readmissions occur, and fewer problems requiring subsequent physician and outpatient services occur.

This is an encouraging finding from Medicare's perspective. First, it would appear that little, if any, gaming of the reimbursement system, through the two approaches to double-dipping discussed earlier, is occurring. That is, since fewer, rather than more, hospital readmissions occur, Medicare is actually saving rather than losing on hospital readmissions for swing-bed patients. The evidence suggests further that whatever ancillary services might be received during the swing-bed stay translate into Medicare savings in terms of subsequent physician, outpatient, and hospital care. It appears that Medicare realizes a 2–3 percent savings per acute care patient per year by virtue of the swing-bed approach.

Program Expenditures

Table 6.8 contains estimates of expenditures for swing-bed care by Medicare and Medicaid. These were estimated for 1985, using survey information on nationwide swing-bed utilization by payer, combined with estimated payment rates by level of care. Total estimated routine care expenditures for Medicare and Medicaid combined were approximately $17.9 million, with $15.8 million paid by Medicare and $2.1 million paid

Table 6.8 Estimated Medicare and Medicaid Expenditures for
Swing-Bed Care, 1985

	Days	Expenditures
Routine care (Medicare)	314,824	$15,814,000
Routine care (Medicaid)	51,359	2,130,000
Ancillary services (Medicare)	314,824	10,279,000

Notes: Survey data for 1985 were utilized to estimate swing-bed days by payer. The average swing-bed hospital participating in the program provided 472 Medicare, 32 Medicaid SNF, and 45 Medicaid ICF swing-bed days. Since 97 percent of the 688 certified swing-bed hospitals as of July 1985 were estimated as providing swing-bed care, the days per hospital were multiplied by 667 to derive the total days by payer.

These expenditure estimates are rounded to the nearest $1,000 and exclude program administration costs incurred by certification and review agencies, fiscal intermediaries, and related organizations, since such costs were found in earlier surveys to be small relative to the total expenditures presented here (see Shaughnessy, Schlenker, et al. 1985).

To estimate routine care expenditures, the average Medicare swing-bed routine rate was derived as the 1985 routine Medicare reimbursement rate by state, weighted by the number of certified swing-bed hospitals in each state. This rate of $50.23 was also used for Medicaid skilled-level swing-bed patient days. The weighted ICF rate of $35.26 was used for the remaining Medicaid days.

Only Medicare ancillary expenditures were estimated since nearly all swing-bed ancillary services are paid by Medicare. The average per diem reimbursement amount of $31.55 from the 1984 cost report sample was inflated to $32.65 for 1985 (using the HCFA inflation factor of 3.5 percent) and multiplied by the estimated number of 1985 Medicare swing-bed days.

by Medicaid. These expenditure estimates do not include program administration costs since analyses of certification, certificate of need, licensure, and fiscal intermediary organizations indicated these costs were inconsequential relative to the total outlays presented in the table. By way of comparison, the estimated Medicare routine swing-bed expenditures represented approximately 2.6 percent of the 1985 Medicare SNF expenditures of $600 million. Medicaid swing-bed expenditures, however, represented less than 0.02 percent of the total Medicaid nursing home expenditures in 1985 of $14.7 billion (Waldo, Levit, and Lazenby 1986).

Since Medicare and Medicaid were found to account for 57 percent of total swing-bed days, the combined 366,183 days for Medicare and Medicaid translate into an estimated 642,426 total days including private-pay days, under the assumption that private pay accounts for 43 percent of total swing-bed days. This figure is slightly less than the lower bound in the range of 750,000 to 1,971,000 long-term care days forecast on the basis of the demonstration program experience in the 1970s. The actual number of swing-bed days in 1985 did not fall into this prediction interval due to a number of factors, not the least of which is that the forecast was premised on the assumption that all rural hospitals, not just hospitals with fewer than 50 beds, would be eligible to participate in the national program. Nonetheless, the prediction interval was regarded as approximate and, from this perspective, not terribly inaccurate. The prediction interval pertained to a point in time when the program would reach its steady state, which was felt to be two years following the implementation of the national program. In effect, the national program began in 1984 in view of the delay in implementing the regulations and the slow start discussed in Chapter 4.

Estimating total program costs including private-pay patients as well as Medicare and Medicaid patients was done in the same manner as for utilization (i.e., assuming private pay accounts for 43 percent of costs). This yielded a total program cost of $31.5 million for 1985. Deflating this to 1978 dollars placed it in the low extreme of the prediction interval of $14.2 to $37.0 million in 1978 dollars—that was forecast on the basis of the demonstration experience in the 1970s. Again, the observed low cost relative to predicted cost is partly due to the difference in eligibility criteria used in the national program from those used for forecasting purposes.

In considering the total cost of swing-bed care to the Medicare program, it is also appropriate to take into consideration the cost that Medicare would have incurred if the swing-bed program had not been implemented. The results presented earlier in Table 6.4 suggest that Medicare saved at least $6.73—and possibly as much as $16.23—per day on the swing-bed program, under the assumption that the days of long-term care provided in swing beds would have been provided in either freestanding or hospital-based SNFs. Under this assumption, the 314,824 Medicare days of swing-bed care shown in Table 6.8 translate into a Medicare savings of between $2.1 and $5.1 million. However, as suggested from the later analysis results in Table 6.7, it is possible that the assumption upon which such savings are premised (i.e., all SNF swing-bed days would translate into SNF days in nursing homes if there were no swing-bed programs) might not be accurate. This is suggested by the finding that total SNF costs for acute care patients discharged from swing-bed hospitals are higher than SNF costs for acute care patients discharged from non-swing-bed hospitals (due to more SNF care provided in swing beds). Table 6.7 shows, however, that acute care patients discharged from non-swing-bed hospitals tend to account for higher home health care costs and higher Part B outpatient/ancillary costs.

In any event, it would appear that a more accurate way to assess total Medicare program savings is by using the final row of Table 6.7, which shows that an annual savings accrues to the Medicare program of

$117 per acute care admission to a swing-bed hospital. As described in the notes to Table 6.8, it was estimated that the total number of hospitals admitting patients to the swing-bed program in 1985 was 667. The average number of acute care admissions for each of these hospitals was 966, yielding a total of 644,322 admissions to swing-bed hospitals in 1985. Even assuming the savings to be substantially less than $117 per acute care admission to swing-bed hospitals, a Medicare savings results in excess of the amount shown in Table 6.8 that Medicare expended on routine care and ancillary care reimbursement for swing-bed care in 1985. It is important to recall that the Medicare savings accrue largely from reductions in rehospitalization and Part B reimbursement. In short, however, it appears that the swing-bed program has very likely paid for itself under Medicare by reducing costs to Medicare in these areas.

CONCLUSIONS ON COST AND COST EFFECTIVENESS

The empirical evidence from the cost component of our national evaluation study led us to conclude that the swing-bed approach is an unusually low-cost means of providing near-acute long-term care in rural communities. The reimbursement rates for swing-bed care in the mid-1980s appeared adequate to cover the incremental cost of providing long-term care in hospital beds. However, with the potential for increasing case-mix intensity in hospital swing beds, such rates should continue to be scrutinized for their adequacy (Silverman 1990). From a hospital perspective, it appears that a break-even point for swing-bed costs versus revenues exists in the range of 2,000–2,500 days of swing-bed care per year. To the extent that a given hospital exceeds this volume of swing-bed care, depending on its state-specific reimbursement rate and other circumstances unique to the hospital, it might be appropriate to consider converting acute care beds to long-term care beds to remain financially solvent with respect to providing long-term care. Nonetheless, except under highly unusual circumstances, the swing-bed approach cannot be regarded as providing a large financial windfall for hospitals. If a hospital is in dire financial straits, it is unlikely that swing beds would represent a solution to its problems.

As noted in the preceding chapter, the swing-bed approach is unusually effective in terms of the quality of care provided to near-acute long-term care patients. Not only were rates of rehospitalization reduced and rates of discharge to independent living increased, but near-acute long-term care patients demonstrated greater improvement in functional outcomes after receiving swing-bed care relative to nursing home care. The fact that the cost of swing-bed care to the Medicare program is less than the cost of nursing home care clearly renders the program cost-effective for providing near-acute long-term care. In fact, this is probably an understatement, since cost analyses suggest the swing-bed approach reduced total costs to the Medicare program by reducing hospitalization rates and the use of outpatient services provided by physicians and ancillary personnel. From this vantage point, it appears that the approach actually saved Medicare more than the entire cost of the swing-bed program.

As a result of the cost and reimbursement analyses conducted as a part of the national evaluation, we recommended that it would be useful to examine the possibility of conditioning swing-bed reimbursement on case-mix intensity, consider combining ancillary and routine care reimbursement in a single payment, and possibly reexamine physician reimbursement policies for near-acute long-term care patients in view of the effectiveness of physician care for such patients. These issues are part of the larger question of what we should do about providing near-acute care in the United States, a topic that is discussed further in the final chapter.

CHAPTER 6 SUMMARY

The evaluation study of the demonstration program in the 1970s found that Medicare and Medicaid reimbursement was sufficient to cover the incremental cost of providing swing-bed care (defining incremental cost to be the add-on cost of providing long-term care in hospital beds that already exist to provide acute care). This was consistent with our earlier finding that Medicare and Medicaid reimbursement based on nursing home rates was slightly higher than this cost. Under the new national program, however, a variety of factors were different. Not only was the program now national in scope, but the tendency to provide near-acute care was even more pronounced, and hospitals very likely had made significant strides in enhancing the effectiveness of long-term care provided in swing beds. If incremental cost of long-term care continued to be reasonably competitive with nursing home cost, Medicare and Medicaid could feasibly save dollars by continuing to encourage hospitals to provide swing-bed care—especially for patients requiring near-acute care.

Although PPS provided incentives for small rural hospitals to participate in the national swing-bed program, it also provided certain incentives to game the new reimbursement system. As a result, cost-related concerns pertained not only to reimbursement for swing-bed care, but to hospital reimbursement as well. The major question in this regard was whether our combined acute care and swing-bed care reimbursement systems were working in an integrated manner for rural hospitals. Related to this was the question of whether the incremental cost of swing-bed care varied according to the volume of care provided and, if so, the ramifications of this for swing-bed hospitals and payers.

Reimbursement rates for Medicare and Medicaid under the swing-bed program are the same as the preceding year's Medicaid reimbursement rates in each state. Thus, the Medicare and Medicaid (if Medicaid is participating in the swing-bed program in a given state) SNF rates for swing-bed care are the same as the prior year's average Medicaid SNF rate in each state. Analogously, the Medicaid ICF rate for swing-bed hospitals is the same as the average Medicaid ICF rate for the preceding year. Medicare pays for ancillary services in the manner it used to pay for ancillary services for hospital care. Namely, it reimburses the hospital for ancillary service costs to swing-bed patients, where such costs are determined by applying the ratio of swing-bed patient ancillary charges over total ancillary charges to total ancillary costs for the hospital.

Three incremental cost estimation procedures based on accounting methods were used. The methods involved similar procedures for estimating the incremental costs of routine and ancillary care. For routine care cost, various overhead cost centers were first allocated to routine care and then to swing-bed care. One incremental cost estimation method involved fewer cost centers than the other two. Only one of the three estimation procedures involved labor costs. This procedure involved the maximum number of cost centers and allocated both labor and nonlabor costs to swing-bed care. It had a different allocation procedure from the other two. The procedure was premised on the assumption that smaller volumes of swing-bed care typically result in very low incremental costs. This assumption was supported by surveys and anecdotal information we obtained from swing-bed hospitals. The three accounting-based cost estimation procedures were also supplemented by statistical or regression-based methods.

Using all three incremental cost estimation methods, we found that average routine care revenues in 1984 exceeded incremental costs for the typical swing-bed hospital. The extent to which revenues exceeded costs, however, varied according to the cost estimation method used. Using the methods that yielded higher costs (which we considered the most appropriate methods), we found that the 1984 average incremental cost for routine care per day in swing-bed hospitals was between $32 and $35—less than the average per day revenue of about $44. After adjusting for a capital and medical education cost carve-out that is part of the Medicare reimbursement approach, we found that the average hospital gained between $8 and $10 per day for routine care under the swing-bed program. Some hospitals, however, lost money on routine care. Magnitudes of gains (or losses) appeared to be related to the volume of care (discussed below), other hospital factors such as occupancy rates, and state-specific reimbursement rates.

Most hospitals tended to do reasonably well under reimbursement for ancillary care. In fact, it is likely that hospitals that lost small amounts of money under routine care reimbursement covered these loses under ancillary reimbursement. The incremental cost estimation methods for ancillary care were similar to those for routine care and involved six major ancillary services: physical therapy, drugs, medical supplies, respiratory therapy, laboratory services, and radiology. We found that the average incremental cost per day for ancillary services was between $18 and $21, compared with an average ancillary care revenue of about $32. Conservatively, we estimated the average excess of per day revenues over incremental costs to be between $10 and $13 per long-term care day.

Although revenues typically exceeded costs for long-term care provided in hospital swing beds, it is important to emphasize that incremental cost was used. Most hospitals continue to feel reimbursement is inadequate since incremental cost is rarely used in determining reimbursement in the health care field. Nevertheless, even if one assumes that Medicare and Medicaid are more than covering the incremental cost of long-term care provided in hospital swing beds, the swing-bed program appears to save Medicare and Medicaid money. If, for example, all Medicare SNF days of care in swing-bed hospitals were provided in hospital-based SNFs, it would have cost the Medicare program $26 more per day in 1984 than under the swing-bed program. Even if Medicare SNF days of swing-bed care were split between hospital-based and free-standing Medicare SNFs, Medicare would have saved $16 per day. Under the unlikely case that all such days of SNF care had been provided in freestanding SNFs, Medicare would have still saved $7 per day. Such per day savings may be lower than Medicare actually realized since urban SNFs (where many swing-bed patients would have been placed) are even more expensive than rural SNFs (whose reimbursement rates were used to calculate the savings). Further, no assumption was made regarding constructing new SNFs, which would have been even more costly in rural communities. However, although Medicare clearly realizes a savings through the swing-bed program, as discussed below, the assumption that all SNF swing-bed days would have been SNF days in a Medicare-certified nursing home is not necessarily valid.

In order to examine whether swing-bed hospitals were gaming the

PPS and swing-bed reimbursement systems, we analyzed Medicare claims data on over 30,000 patients discharged from swing-bed and non-swing-bed comparison hospitals in 1985. We found that total Medicare costs were less for patients discharged from swing-bed hospitals than from non-swing-bed hospitals. The savings that accrued to Medicare was largely due to a substitution of swing-bed care for both subsequent acute care and physician/outpatient care occurring after discharge. Thus, on the basis of the quality-of-care findings from the preceding chapter, it is likely that improved rehabilitation—and discharge home because of such rehabilitation—by swing-bed hospitals resulted in fewer hospital admissions and fewer problems requiring subsequent physician and outpatient services. This is desirable from Medicare's perspective because it confirms that little if any gaming of the reimbursement system is occurring. Fewer, rather than more, hospital readmissions are occurring because of swing-bed care, and Medicare is, in fact, saving rather than losing on hospital readmissions for swing-bed patients. In addition, the ancillary services that are received during the swing-bed stay apparently translate into Medicare savings in terms of subsequent physician, outpatient, and hospital care. In all, it appears that a 2–3 percent savings per acute care patient per year accrues to Medicare through the swing-bed approach.

Our analysis revealed an increase in incremental cost per day as a function of the total number of days of long-term care provided by a swing-bed hospital. This is in keeping with the expectation that the more long-term care days a hospital provides in swing beds, the more likely it is to incur higher unit costs attributable to new staff costs, maintenance costs, and so forth. If a fairly minimal amount of swing-bed care were provided, it would very likely not incur new costs in such areas. Our calculations showed that a break-even threshold exists between 2,000 and 2,500 days of long-term care for the average swing-bed hospital. If a small hospital provides more days of swing-bed care than this, it should consider converting hospital beds to distinct-part SNF beds for which reimbursement is more generous than swing-bed reimbursement based on incremental cost. The precise threshold, of course, depends on an individual hospital's cost structure and the Medicare and Medicaid reimbursement rates for the state in which the hospital is located.

Total Medicare and Medicaid expenditures on the swing-bed program in 1985 were approximately $28 million. An estimated 642,000 days of swing-bed care, including private-pay days as well as Medicare and Medicaid days, were provided in hospital swing beds in 1985. This figure is slightly less than the lower bound in the range of 750,000 to 1.9 million long-term care days forecast on the basis of the demonstration program experience in the 1970s. Analogously, deflating the total expenditure for Medicare and Medicaid on swing-bed care to 1978 dollars places it in the low extreme of the prediction interval of $14.2 to $37.0 million in 1978 dollars forecast on the basis of the demonstration experience in the 1970s. Swing-bed expenditures represented approximately 3 percent of the 1985 Medicare SNF expenditures; Medicaid swing-bed expenditures represented less than 0.02 percent of total Medicaid nursing home expenditures in 1985. Thus, swing-bed care is presently a relatively small component of our long-term care delivery system.

Since an analysis of Medicare claims data showed that not all Medicare swing-bed SNF days necessarily translate into nursing home SNF days (i.e., some translate into home health care, others into reduced hospital stays, and so on), it appears that the most accurate way to assess total Medicare savings under the swing-bed program is by examining the longitudinal cost per hospital admission to swing-bed hospitals versus non-swing-bed hospitals. Even assuming the savings to be substantially less than the estimated $117 per acute care admission to swing-bed hospitals, a Medicare savings results in excess of the total Medicare expenditures on routine care and ancillary care reimbursement for swing-bed care in 1985. Thus, it appears that the swing-bed program has paid for itself under Medicare by lowering costs through reductions in rehospitalizations and physician reimbursement after discharge.

Because the swing-bed approach is effective in terms of the quality of care provided to near-acute long-term care patients, and because it is less costly than SNF care for the Medicare program, we have concluded that the program is cost-effective. We recommended that Medicare examine the possibility of incorporating patient needs or case-mix intensity into reimbursement for swing-bed care, that it consider combining ancillary and routine care reimbursement into a single payment, and that it possibly reexamine physician reimbursement policies for near-acute care patients in view of the effectiveness of physician care for these types of patients. Overall, the remarkable success of the swing-bed program raises the question of what we should do in providing near-acute care in the United States.

PART **III**

Policy Issues, Related Topics, and Recommendations

Recent Developments Pertinent to Shaping Near-Acute Care Policy

AN OVERVIEW OF THE CURRENT SITUATION

The 1980s probably brought the most pronounced set of changes of any decade in our history in terms of increased patient care needs or case-mix intensity in the hospital, nursing home, and home health care fields. This was in part due to the implementation of Medicare's prospective payment system (PPS), which substantially influenced the way hospital care was provided in the United States in the early to mid-1980s. The changes in hospital care in turn affected the types of patients admitted to and cared for in various subacute long-term care settings (the term *subacute* is used here to mean any type of care that is less intense than acute hospital care). As hospital stays shortened, patients with more near-acute care needs were admitted to various types of long-term care settings, in turn causing shifts in admission and discharge patterns for other types of long-term care providers. The need for near-acute care services became clearer and more pronounced.

At the same time, other important policy, programmatic, and research developments provided further information about what might and might not work in the near-acute long-term care field. An increased awareness of the differences between near-acute and traditional long-term care was manifest (although the term *near-acute long-term care* was not used). Geriatrics and gerontology, subfields of the medical profession and social/health care fields, respectively, continued to expand their horizons, dealing with a range of patient needs, including near-acute care. Various programs for assessing and treating geriatric patients yielded information on essential aspects of providing near-acute care. Ongoing provider experimentation is continuing to yield relevant information in this regard. Lessons learned from the passage and repeal of the Medicare Catastrophic Coverage Act of 1988 bear remembering. In the late 1980s, the national swing-bed program was expanded to larger hospitals in rural areas; the precise ramifications of this change for near-acute care will probably not be clear until the mid-1990s.

NATIONAL CHANGES IN THE CARE NEEDS
OF LONG-TERM CARE PATIENTS

Precipitating Policy Changes in the Late 1970s and 1980s

A number of initiatives in the late 1970s and early 1980s brought about significant changes in the supply and orientation of providers of long-term care. Some of these initiatives were briefly mentioned in Chapter 3. For example, the movement to deinstitutionalize long-term care was manifest in newly implemented Medicaid initiatives in several states by the early 1980s (Weissert, Cready, and Pawelak 1988; Kemper, Applebaum, and Harrigan 1987; Hughes 1985). These initiatives were often characterized by a strong preadmission screening component for nursing home residents intended to divert potential nursing home admissions to home- and community-based care programs under Section 2176 of the Omnibus Budget Reconciliation Act of 1981 (OBRA 1981, P.L. 97-35). They were intended to reduce nursing home placement for patients who were only mildly debilitated in terms of their functional needs. If successful, such programs would therefore have the effect of intensifying case mix in nursing homes by the mid-1980s by increasing the proportion of patients with moderate-to-intense functional needs.

Second, accompanying the efforts on the part of state Medicaid programs to promote home- and community-based care, the supply of Medicare-certified home health care providers grew substantially between 1980 and 1988, increasing by slightly over 100 percent (HCFA 1989c). Increases in Medicare-certified home health care occurred largely in the early to mid-1980s; the use of certified home health care stabilized during the late 1980s in most locations. The growth in Medicare home health care utilization for skilled nursing patients was almost exponential, from approximately 500,000 visits in 1978 to 1.3 million in 1982 (Sankar, Newcomer, and Wood 1986). Use of home health care within 60 days of hospital discharge rose from 9.1 percent in 1981 to 14.1 percent in 1983, a 55 percent increase (Gornick and Hall 1988). This increase in home health care utilization was due in part to provisions in the Omnibus Budget Reconciliation Act of 1980 (OBRA 1980, P.L. 96-499) that eliminated the 100-visit limit, the Part A prior hospitalization requirement, the Part B deductible, and the requirement of state licensure for Medicare certification of home health agencies (Ruther and Helbing 1988). Medicare home health care played an increasingly important role throughout the 1980s in providing long-term care to patients with near-acute care needs who could be treated in an independent living environment.

Third, the ripple effects—perhaps more appropriately the shock waves—of PPS reverberated from the hospital field to the long-term care field for the better part of the 1980s. The incentives to discharge patients from hospital care after shorter stays and with potentially stronger postacute care needs gave rise to the oft-used phrase that patients were now discharged "quicker and sicker" (U.S. Congress, House 1989). In the mid-1980s, just a short time after PPS had been implemented, we had only anecdotal information from nursing homes, home health agencies, and other types of long-term care providers suggesting that the case mix of their patients, residents, or clients seemed to be intensifying in various ways. The contention was made by care providers that resource needs of long-term care patients were increasing because of PPS (Lyles 1986; Seifer 1987; Helbing and Keene 1989). The extent to which this was occurring systematically, rather than sporadically or in isolated locations, was unknown in the mid- to late 1980s, however.

Fourth, with changes taking place due to the diversion of patients from nursing homes, increases in home health care, and shorter hospital stays, questions about quality and effectiveness of long-term care naturally intensified. Were patients going to be rehospitalized more often because of the quicker and sicker incentives imposed on the acute care field by PPS? Would long-term care providers be overtaxed in their ability to provide adequate care to patients being discharged quicker and sicker from hospitals? Would the nursing home diversion programs set up in various states be detrimental to patients who should be in nursing homes but may have been diverted by well-intended but potentially flawed preadmission screening programs? Peer review organizations (PROs) had been set up as an accompaniment of PPS to monitor both utilization and quality of care (Peer Review Improvement Act of 1982, contained in the Tax Equity and Fiscal Responsibility Act of 1982, P.L. 97-248). Their charge was no small challenge. In fact, it was massive. Our rather minimal knowledge of how to measure and assure quality inhibited PROs from hitting the ground running—to say nothing of being able to make even moderate progress over a period of several years.

Empirical Findings on Case-Mix Changes in Different Provider Settings

At the same time our research center was carrying out the national swing-bed evaluation, we were conducting a longitudinal study to monitor change in case mix in selected long-term care provider settings during the 1980s. The findings from this HCFA-funded study are summarized in the following discussion along with relevant findings from the work of others.

For purposes of this discussion, and in keeping with the terminology introduced in the first chapter, *traditional nursing homes* are defined as Medicaid-certified (not necessarily Medicare-certified) nursing homes that provide care to relatively few Medicare patients. Traditional nursing homes have a Medicare use rate, the percentage of patient days covered by Medicare, ranging from 0 to 5 percent, typically averaging 1 to 2 percent. The term *Medicare nursing home* here refers to a Medicare-certified nursing home that has a reasonably substantial proportion of its patient days covered by Medicare, typically with a Medicare use rate exceeding 15 percent. Thus, this definition of Medicare nursing homes precludes the majority of Medicare-certified nursing homes that provide but small amounts of Medicare SNF care. *Certified home health agencies* are defined to be Medicare-certified home health agencies with Medicare use rates between 30 and 95 percent, averaging approximately 75 percent. Further details on these definitions and study findings are available elsewhere (Shaughnessy and Kramer 1990; Shaughnessy, Kramer, et al. 1987).

Case-Mix Changes in Traditional Nursing Homes during the 1980s. In the HCFA-funded study, a general trend toward increased functional dependency was observed in traditional nursing home residents. In such facilities, residents were characterized by increasing dependence in activities of daily living (ADLs), instrumental activities of daily living (IADLs), and various chronic long-term care problems. Such disabilities included, but were not restricted to, dressing, eating, toileting, incontinence, speech impairments, and diabetes. Aggregate case-mix indicators supported the relatively pronounced increase in the intensity of functional and chronic long-term care problems. This increasing functional and chronic care case-mix intensity in traditional nursing homes during the 1980s was attributable to a stronger increase in the prevalence of such problems for Medicaid patients rather than non-Medicaid patients.

The results showed little increase in the intensity of near-acute care needs for patients in traditional nursing homes. Selected indicators of near-acute care, such as the percentage of bedfast patients and the percentage of patients with orthopnea or who required oxygen, demonstrated some degree of increase between 1982 and 1986. However, other near-acute indicators did not increase over time, such as the percentage of tube-fed patients, insulin-requiring diabetics, patients with recent surgery, and those with diastolic hypertension.

Further evidence of this case-mix trend in traditional nursing homes comes from the 1985 National Nursing Home Survey, which showed that functional disabilities of traditional nursing home patients increased between 1977 and 1985 (Seksenski 1987). Not only are traditional long-term care patients now more dependent in their need for various types of care, especially functional care, but hospitalization rates for nursing home patients have been steadily increasing. Between 1977 and 1985, the hospitalization rate for elderly patients discharged alive from nursing homes increased from 39 to 50 percent nationally. In some locations, the increase in the proportion of nursing home patients that are hospitalized appears to be even more substantial. In Wisconsin, for example, hospitalization rates for Medicaid patients admitted to nursing homes rose from 15 to 26 percent between 1982 and 1984 (Sager, Leventhal, and Fasterling 1987). Lewis et al. (1990) found that patients (admitted to 47 skilled nursing facilities in southern California) with a prior history of nursing home care were far more likely to have poorer health status and be readmitted to hospital care in 1984 than in 1980. Increased hospitalization of nursing home residents is undoubtedly due in part to the increased case-mix intensity discussed above. But it may also reflect an inadequacy of our current long-term care delivery system to respond properly to the increased care needs of patients.

Case-Mix Changes in Medicare Nursing Homes in the 1980s. Medicare patients in Medicare nursing homes exhibited what appears to be a pronounced effect of PPS in terms of increased near-acute case-mix intensity. Important near-acute tracer conditions such as tube-feeding, being bedfast, severe orthopnea or the need for oxygen, IV catheters, near-acute cardiovascular problems, congestive heart failure, and diastolic hypertension all reflected relatively pronounced increases in prevalence rates between 1983 and 1986 for Medicare patients in Medicare nursing homes. Aggregate ADL case-mix indicators revealed virtually no change, however, in terms of the prevalence of ADL dependency for Medicare patients in such nursing homes over this time period.

Although the total volume of Medicare SNF admissions (per Medicare enrollee) remained fairly constant from 1981 through 1987, consistent with the above-mentioned changes, the proportion of Medicare SNF admissions from acute care hospitals rose considerably over this period (Latta and Keene 1989). During the later part of the 1980s, changes in the SNF coverage guidelines and the Catastrophic Coverage Act of 1988 (P.L. 100-360) increased Medicare SNF utilization considerably, bringing about what appeared to be a temporary case-mix change in Medicare nursing homes in 1989.

The fairly substantial case-mix changes for near-acute problems were more pronounced for Medicare patients than non-Medicare patients in Medicare nursing homes. While certain near-acute problem indicators demonstrated increased prevalence for non-Medicare patients between 1983 and 1986, the increase in near-acute care needs for Medicare patients in such facilities was considerably greater.

Case-Mix Changes in Medicare Home Health Agencies during the 1980s. Disability levels for ADLs and IADLs intensified between the early and mid-1980s for patients under the care of Medicare-certified home health agencies. Certain near-acute problems, such as tube-feeding, being bedfast, orthopnea, oxygen requirements, and insulin-dependent diabetes, also became more prevalent for home health patients over this period. In general, increased dependency in functioning as well as a modest increase in prevalence of near-acute problems characterized the case-mix changes in home health agencies between 1982 and 1986. Nearly all increases that occurred in the intensity of home health agency case mix were due to changes occurring in Medicare home health case mix. In fact, functional disabilities for non-Medicare home health patients exhibited a decrease in prevalence over this period. Non-Medicare patients did, however, show a mild increase in certain near-acute problems. Nonetheless, the percentage of home health patients admitted from hospitals as well as the percentage (but not the number) of Medicare patients decreased over this time, since the total number of home health care patients increased.

Case-Mix Changes in Acute Care Hospitals during the 1980s. The changes in acute care hospital case mix that occurred between the early and mid-1980s are now well documented (Guterman et al. 1988). First, lengths of stay decreased for all payers, with Medicare lengths of stay decreasing more substantially than non-Medicare stays. Second, generally speaking, hospital case mix intensified during the 1980s in terms of resource requirements. This is demonstrated in the aggregate by a national increase in the case-mix acuity index used by Medicare to reflect resource consumption needs of hospital patients (Helbing and Keene 1989; Carter and Ginsburg 1985; Guterman et al. 1988; Morrisey, Sloan, and Valvona 1988). Most physicians and nurses, as well as other hospital staff, generally agree that, while hospital occupancy rates dropped over this time, the average patient admitted to an acute care hospital in the mid- to late 1980s had greater resource needs than the average patient admitted to acute care in the late 1970s and early 1980s—apparently because certain types of patients with more mild or less urgent care needs are simply not hospitalized as frequently as during the early 1980s (Conklin and Houchens 1987; Liu and Manton 1988).

Causes and Effects of Changing Resource Needs of Long-Term Care Patients

PPS Impacts. Although it is not appropriate to conclude that the changes long-term care providers were experiencing in the 1980s were due exclusively to PPS, there is no doubt PPS was instrumental in bringing about several of these changes. The effects of PPS on traditional nursing homes appeared to be indirect. While the intensity of functional and chronic long-term care problems increased in such facilities, changes in near-acute problems were minimal. The increases in chronic care case mix in traditional facilities probably had as much to do with intensified Medicaid preadmission screening programs, home- and community-based care programs, moratoria on additional nursing home beds in many states, and a general movement to divert nursing home admissions to noninstitutional settings, as it did with PPS.

The case-mix changes that characterized Medicare nursing homes reflected a more direct PPS impact. A substantial increase in near-acute case-mix intensity after PPS was found in nursing homes with Medicare use rates that averaged approximately 25 percent. Unlike the case-mix changes in more traditional nursing homes, the increases in prevalence of typical long-term care problems and ADLs were relatively minimal in such Medicare SNFs. These types of nursing homes gravitated even more strongly toward near-acute care than was the case prior to PPS, very likely diverting patients with no near-acute care needs to traditional nursing homes.

This diversion of patients with less intense near-acute care needs probably occurred as a result of several concurrent factors. For example, it likely resulted from physician judgment of the capability of various nursing homes available to care for a given patient, changing admission policies of nursing homes, and other patient-specific circumstances. Regardless, the findings suggest such diversions took place with relatively great frequency in the mid- to late 1980s. The fact that the patients diverted apparently had less near-acute but possibly stronger ADL/chronic long-term care needs partly accounted for the increased intensity in functional and chronic problems in traditional nursing homes. Another significant case-mix impact of PPS appeared to have been on providers of home health care. Not only did several near-acute case-mix indicators increase between 1982 and 1986 for Medicare-certified home health agencies in the study, but also functional and more chronic long-term care problems increased even more substantially, almost uniformly.

The moderate increase in near-acute case-mix intensity and the substantial increase in functional care needs for home health patients was due almost exclusively to increased case-mix intensity for Medicare rather than non-Medicare patients.

Combined Effects of Medicaid Policy, PPS, and Increased Home Health Supply. The increased resource needs associated with physical/ADL functioning for home health agencies were very likely a combined effect of PPS and the efforts of Medicaid programs to divert some types of long-term care patients from nursing homes. The national movement by Medicaid programs to tighten preadmission screening for nursing homes and to increase functional support services available in the community had the effect of diverting selected potential Medicaid nursing home admissions to home health care. Increased availability of personal care and homemaker services in the community through Medicaid and other programs, in combination with intermittent skilled nursing visits covered by Medicare, expanded the supply of home health care available to patients with greater functional needs. Under earlier Medicaid practices, such patients might have been institutionalized, although they had fewer functional disabilities than most other nursing home patients. Nonetheless, when retained in the community and provided home care, they would tend to be more functionally disabled than the typical home care patient. Thus, it is likely that there was some substitution, at least at the margin, of Medicare home health care for Medicaid nursing home care. This would have the combined effect that was observed: An increase would occur in the ADL or functional care case-mix intensity of traditional nursing homes (which previously admitted less functionally dependent patients), along with an increase in the functional care case-mix intensity of home health agencies (which previously admitted patients who were minimally dependent in ADLs).

The proliferation of home health agencies over this same period and a decrease in the percentage of home health patients admitted from hospitals at first suggests the possibility of overuse of Medicare home health services relative to the pre-PPS period. However, this hypothesis is questionable since the case-mix intensity of Medicare home health patients increased over the same period. It would appear, despite the increase in the number of home health providers and the decrease in the number of home health admissions from acute care hospitals, that home health agencies encountered a general increase in the medical, skilled nursing, and functional needs of Medicare patients.

The stabilization of—and, in some areas, moderate decrease in—case-mix intensity for private-pay home health patients was probably a function of the increased supply of home health providers. On the one hand, the impact of PPS may have been sufficiently strong to increase the case-mix intensity of Medicare patients uniformly in home health agencies that existed prior to PPS (despite the large number of agencies that were certified since PPS took effect). However, it also appears that the increase in total supply perhaps saturated the private-pay market for home health care.

Reimbursement and Quality Issues. While no comprehensive study was conducted to examine the extent to which reimbursement (Medicare or Medicaid) was commensurate with case-mix changes over this period, four points are noteworthy. First, the case-mix changes in traditional nursing homes pertained predominantly to Medicaid and private-pay patients, and therefore fall under the rubric of state-directed reimbursement policy.

Second, a number of state Medicaid programs throughout the country either have been or are considering reimbursing nursing homes on the basis of case mix. While reimbursement policies, procedures, and amounts vary considerably from state to state, the recognition that case mix should somehow be taken into consideration in reimbursing providers of nursing home care is now reasonably widespread (Foley 1989).

Third, unlike Medicaid reimbursement in most states and hospital reimbursement nationally, Medicare continues to reimburse for SNF care on the basis of costs incurred by SNFs. Nevertheless, such reimbursement is cost-based only up to limits. When a facility reaches these limits (which are separate for hospital-based and freestanding nursing homes), no additional reimbursement is available. An analysis of precisely how many SNFs have exceeded these cost limits, and the reasons why, has not yet been undertaken. It would appear that the relationship between reimbursement, case mix, and quality requires more systematic scrutiny in the long-term care field than it has thus far received nationally. (Medicare is presently undertaking a demonstration project to experiment with case-mix reimbursement for SNF care.) As a corollary, we need a comprehensive analysis of the manner in which we provide, regulate, and pay for near-acute long-term care in view of the substantial changes that have taken place in this critical component of the long-term care field in the 1980s.

Fourth, in view of the documented increases in resource needs and hospitalization rates for long-term patients in the 1980s and relatively few changes in reimbursement policy, it is not clear whether current reimbursement policies are the most appropriate (in fact, they may be acceptable, we simply do not know). Thus, we must investigate whether the quality of care in long-term care settings is adequate for the newer, hard-to-care-for types of patients now found in several such settings.

THE NEED TO ADDRESS NEAR-ACUTE CARE

Subacute Care and Transitional Care

Because of changes in case mix and related factors, providers throughout the United States were confronted with what subsequently became the subacute care and transitional care movements. These two movements were similar, differing substantively in certain ways, but often only in terms of semantics. They arose largely because hospitals found it difficult to place certain types of postacute patients in long-term care settings. They also stimulated interest in the issue of intensified case mix in nursing homes. Some of the nursing home case-mix reimbursement systems that had been established in the late 1970s and early 1980s—for example, the trailblazing systems in states such as West Virginia, Ohio, Illinois, and Maryland (Grimaldi and Jazwiecki 1987; Foley et al. 1984)— did not appear to satisfactorily take into consideration that the post-PPS patients of the middle and late 1980s often had stronger medical/ skilled nursing needs or rehabilitation needs than pre-PPS nursing home patients.

The term *subacute care* was initially introduced in some circles to mean any type of long-term care that is less medically intense than acute care (e.g., nursing home care, home health care). To some extent, this usage persists. For example, the Prospective Payment Assessment Commission defines subacute care in the hospital setting as "care provided to patients who do not meet established criteria for medically necessary acute care" (ProPAC 1988). The American Hospital Association (AHA) tends to use the term in a manner that is almost synonymous with SNF care. Most frequently, however, the use of the term is more restrictive. It is usually thought of as that level of care needed by a patient who does not require acute hospital care, but who does require more intensive nursing than is normally provided in a SNF (Grim 1989; Timmreck 1989). For example, the Ohio Health Department defines subacute patients as "no longer needing acute care, requiring 3.5 or more hours of skilled nursing care by a licensed nurse per day, and requiring two or more procedures that can only be performed by a licensed nurse or certified therapist" (Trisel 1988).

Other state Medicaid programs explored and developed reimbursement guidelines for subacute care, providing additional reimbursement for special types of patients (Lipson and Thomas 1986). For example, California defined the subacute level of care as "that level of care needed by a patient who does not require acute care but who requires more intensive licensed skilled nursing care than is normally provided in a skilled nursing facility" (Title 22, California Administrative Code,

Section 51124.5, Subacute Level of Care; Lipson and Thomas 1986, Attachment 1). The California definition went on to state:

> . . . to be eligible for the subacute level of care, a patient's condition shall require all of the following as determined by the patient's attending physician and as approved by the appropriate Medi-Cal field office medical consultant or equivalent authorizing agent, who is responsible for authorizing the level of care:
>
> (1) Physician visits medically required at least twice weekly during the first month and a minimum of at least once every week thereafter.
>
> (2) Twenty-four hour access via written agreement(s) to services only available in a general acute hospital.
>
> (3) Special medical equipment and supplies, such as ventilators, which are in addition to those listed in [an administrative code title].
>
> (4) Twenty-four hour licensed nursing care, including treatment procedure(s) during all three shifts which can be performed only by a registered nurse or licensed vocational nurse.
>
> (5) Administration of three or more treatment procedures as provided for in [an administrative manual].

At the same time, transitional care was evolving nationally, largely in response to PPS. The term *transitional care,* sometimes used synonymously with subacute care, arose from the postacute nature of such care and the need to provide care that would assist in the transition from acute care to other modalities of care. Upon discharge from an acute care hospital, a postacute patient now tends to need more acute care–like services than before, possibly requiring an institutional stay to receive such services. Such a stay may not have been necessary prior to PPS due to the more extended nature of hospital stays (Lewin/ICF 1988; Mitchell 1989; Polich, Secord, and Parker 1986). Nonetheless, the phrase *transitional care* is not always used to connote medically intense care. One of its broader definitions is provided by the AHA (1989), which defines transitional care as care provided in the hospital to patients who should be discharged from the hospital to other (difficult-to-find) care settings. This includes care for largely elderly patients who require some types of near-acute services. However, transitional care is by no means limited to the elderly population. It also pertains to persons with AIDS, technology-dependent children, substance abusers, homeless people, and ventilator-dependent patients, who also find it difficult to obtain transitional care. This broader definition of transitional care is sometimes referred to as "alternative level of care" (ALC) (Eastwood 1990). Others, however, refer to transitional care as care provided to patients who are similar to acute care patients in their care needs, but who might be receiving institutional care in any one of a variety of settings, including nursing homes, home health settings, rehabilitation hospitals, and short-term general hospitals.

Swing-Bed Care and Near-Acute Care

As a number of fragmented policies regarding subacute care and transitional care were being patchworked together at the state level, the swing-bed program was expanding in rural areas throughout the United States. Interestingly, the very type of subacute or transitional care that was the focus of concern in many states, especially in major metropolitan areas, seemed to be naturally evolving in swing-bed hospitals in rural communities. While in metropolitan areas, freestanding nursing homes were often unwilling to admit patients with substantial 24-hour nursing needs (Oregon Association of Hospitals 1986) and hospital-based nursing homes often had a high rate of occupancy due to patients with transitional care or subacute care needs (Holahan et al. 1988; Dubay and Cohen 1988), rural communities in which swing-bed hospitals were located had developed a cost-effective model for providing such care. The need for ancillary and skilled nursing services for such subacute care patients at times exceeded the service capacity of nursing homes, resulting in discharge from nursing home care and admission to an acute care hospital. Yet, when such patients were placed in hospital swing beds, the availability of these services usually satisfied the patient's needs without having to admit to acute care. Equally important, care coordination (involving different providers of care) was better in swing-bed hospitals since the patient's acute care records, history, and staff providing acute care were readily accessible to staff providing long-term care. In fact, patients often remained in the same bed when transferred to long-term care in swing beds, and long-term care the staff at times included some of the same staff who had provided acute care.

The phraseology associated with transitional care and subacute care arose for a variety of reasons. In many ways, the spirit of these terms connotes the reasonable proximity of intensive services to meet acute care–like needs. The term *near-acute care* has been introduced in this book to more directly connote the care needs of such patients. Since subacute care has a variety of definitions in different states and can refer to any type of care that is less intense than acute care, it is not sufficiently descriptive for our purposes here. In addition, *transitional care* typically refers to postacute care and has come to refer to types of postacute care other than near-acute care. Most reimbursement for near-acute long-term care patients is provided, albeit cost-ineffectively for several types of patients, under the current Medicare long-term care benefit. Thus, improved methods of care and enhanced cost effectiveness of care for such patients should be of interest to Medicare policy-makers.

Quality of Near-Acute Care in the Context of Quality of Long-Term Care

The significant changes in resource needs for long-term care patients occurring in the early 1980s was accompanied by a growing concern about the ability of long-term care providers to adequately meet such needs. This was superimposed on the already entrenched concerns about nursing home care and, to some extent, home health care that continued through the late 1970s and early 1980s (IOM 1986; American Bar Association 1986; Moss and Halamandaris 1977; Harrington and Grant 1988; U.S. Congress, Senate 1986a, 1986b). Earlier concerns were based more on unmet needs of traditional long-term care patients, but it became apparent that attention was now warranted in terms of the adequacy of our entire long-term care delivery system from the dual perspective of quality of and access to care.

The aforementioned study conducted by the Institute of Medicine to examine nursing home care resulted in recommendations that dealt predominantly with traditional long-term care, not necessarily the unique concerns of near-acute long-term care. Therefore, the resulting nursing home reform initiatives (contained in OBRA 1987, P.L. 100-203) and their resident-centered orientation should assist over the course of time in monitoring and rectifying some of the quality-of-care and quality-of-life problems in traditional nursing homes. Especially note-worthy in these OBRA 1987 long-term care facility and home health care regulations were the training requirements for nurses aides and home-maker aides. These requirements resulted from the now reasonably widespread recognition that nurses aides and homemaker aides must have adequate training and be properly credentialed to ensure that func-tional care and a variety of types of support care are properly provided.

Despite more stringent requirements for enhanced provider capa-bilities that will likely be promulgated throughout the 1990s, we still have considerable ground to cover to ensure that long-term care is well provided, or at least adequately monitored so that we can make neces-sary corrections and changes. Issues such as proper placement in an institutional versus noninstitutional setting are far from resolved. Some research findings now available suggest that certain types of patients should not be cared for at home unless home caregivers are knowledge-able about patient needs. For example, a study of outcomes found that incontinent patients and patients with impaired ability to transfer (e.g., from bed to chair, from bed or chair to the bathroom) have better outcomes (in terms of improved patient status) when treated in a nursing home rather than in a home care setting (Shaughnessy, Kramer, et al. 1987). While such studies do not point unequivocally to which types of long-term care patients should or should not be institutionalized, they are beginning to provide information on what settings appear to be more successful for different types of patients. They also suggest what must be done to compensate if a potentially less effective setting is chosen over a more effective setting for a given patient.

FORMATIVE EVENTS AND PRACTICES IN THE EVOLUTION OF NEAR-ACUTE LONG-TERM CARE

Reduced Hospitalization through Improved Long-Term Care

It is apparent that patient needs for near-acute care intensified substantially during the 1980s throughout the United States. It is also apparent that most near-acute care is provided to patients that were recently discharged from hospitals. We are now more keenly aware of the critical portals represented by hospital discharge and discharge from near-acute care as entry points to our traditional long-term care system. And we are now learning that well-provided near-acute care (and traditional long-term care) can have a substantial impact on lessening the need for and utilization of both acute care and long-term care services. A number of innovations and ideas have been recently advanced on how to improve postacute care and how to improve rehabilitation for geriatric patients (Vladeck and Alfano 1987; Kemp, Brummel-Smith, and Ramsdell 1990). A wide array of approaches have also been developed for assessing the functional needs of geriatric patients (Applegate, Blass, and Williams 1990). The original Medicare extended care facility benefit, implemented in the late 1960s, was premised on the hypothesis that hospital care could be lessened if extended care facilities existed to provide postacute extended care. The significant increases in acute care *and* long-term care in the late 1960s, however, were considered to be a refutation of this hypothesis. Until recently, many thought that relatively little substitution of long-term care services for acute care services was possible. This dictum is now being seriously challenged by an increasing number of providers and researchers.

For example, swing-bed hospitals have obviously been successful in substantially reducing rehospitalization for long-term care patients through the provision of high-quality near-acute care. The Robert Wood Johnson Foundation's teaching nursing home program, which was targeted on reducing acute care hospitalizations for nursing home patients, was also successful in lowering hospital episodes for traditional long-term care patients (Shaughnessy, Kramer, and Hittle 1990). While the evidence remains somewhat mixed, it appears that certain types of providers, such as geriatric nurse practitioners, may be effective in bringing about a reduction in hospital admissions of nursing home patients (Kane, Garrard, Buchanan, et al. 1989; Kane, Garrard, Skay, et al. 1989; Kane, Kane, et al. 1988; Buchanan et al. 1989; Master et al. 1980). Other select long-term care programs, discussed later in this chapter, have also successfully reduced hospitalization for long-term care patients (Zimmer et al. 1988; Rubenstein et al. 1984).

It appears that at least three attributes have usually characterized programs in which the provision of long-term care services, be they near-acute care services or traditional long-term care services, have successfully reduced hospitalization. First, and perhaps foremost, is the more integrated provider-team approach that exists in these environments. Closer communication on patient's needs and requisite services among different types of providers, including nurses, physicians, specialized therapists, social workers, and nurses aides, has generally occurred. Second, a more comprehensive approach to assessment and reassessment of the care needs of individual patients or residents has taken place. Third, increased physician involvement or supervision often accompanies such programs. These three commonalities—an integrated team approach to providing long-term care, a comprehensive approach to assessing and monitoring patient needs, and increased physician involvement—therefore would appear to be essential ingredients in assuring the quality of long-term care, including quality in the increasingly important field of near-acute long-term care. Other research points to additional essential features.

Research on Geriatric Assessment and Treatment

Inpatient Geriatric Assessment and Treatment. Termed *geriatric evaluation units (GEUs)* or *geriatric assessment centers (GACs)*, a number of inpatient programs exist or have been initiated to comprehensively assess care needs—at times focusing on near-acute care—of potential long-term care patients in Europe, Canada, and more recently, in some locations in the United States (Read and O'Brien 1989; Williamson 1989; Williams et al. 1987; Chekryn and Roos 1979; Rubenstein, Abrass, and Kane 1981). The evidence available on such units, which at times are accompanied by a companion inpatient (and, sometimes, outpatient) program emphasizing rehabilitation care, provides at least some cause for optimism. The units typically emphasize integrated assessment and monitoring of the long-term care needs of geriatric patients, often providing short-term rehabilitation care for patients requiring such care. In those GEUs or GACs where rehabilitation care is also provided as part of their care program, a team approach to monitoring progress, reevaluating care needs, and providing care is still a key ingredient of the overall approach.

Some geriatric assessment and treatment programs that focus on near-acute long-term care represent a formalization of what seems to have happened naturally, but certainly less comprehensively, under the national swing-bed program in rural hospitals. Essentially, a determination of care needs is made for geriatric patients after a relatively short stay in a near-acute care setting in these types of GEUs and GACs. If, after a comprehensive assessment, it is determined that the patient requires a reasonably intensive rehabilitation program, it can be provided in either the same setting or a companion program integrated with the GEU or GAC. Otherwise, the patient may be referred to another long-term care setting (possibly home) in accord with his or her needs. Just as with swing-bed hospitals where some exceptions exist (i.e., some swing-bed hospitals tend to provide longer-term chronic care), some GEUs and GACs also provide chronic care to patients whose stay is longer in such units. Regardless, the hallmark of geriatric assessment is a thorough and rigorous assessment of care needs, often of near-acute care patients, prior to establishing a program of long-term care (Schuman et al. 1978; Lefton, Bonstelle, and Frengley 1983; Rubenstein, Rhee, and Kane 1982; Morishita et al. 1989).

As stated by Solomon (1988, p. 2,452):

> Comprehensive geriatric assessment is defined as a multidisciplinary evaluation in which the multiple problems of older persons are uncovered, described, and explained, if possible, and in which resources and strengths of the person are cataloged, need for services assessed, and a coordinated care plan developed to focus interventions on the person's problems. The goals of comprehensive geriatric assessment are (1) to improve diagnostic accuracy, (2) to guide the selection of interventions to restore or preserve health, (3) to recommend an optimal environment for care, (4) to predict outcomes, and (5) to monitor clinical change over time.

This definition and the stated goals resulted from a conference sponsored by the National Institutes of Health on geriatric assessment methods for clinical decision making. The conference statement indicated the following (Solomon 1988, p. 2,452):

> Comprehensive geriatric assessment generally includes evaluation of the patient in several domains, most commonly the physical, mental, social, economic, functional, and environmental characteristics. . . . It is conducted by a core team that consists, at a minimum, of a physician, nurse, and social worker, each with special expertise in caring for older people.

Frequently, a psychiatrist is a member of the core team. Other participating professions may include audiology, clinical psychology, dentistry, nutrition, occupational therapy, optometry, pharmacy, physical therapy, podiatry, and speech pathology. . . . Support from other medical disciplines, such as neurology, ophthalmology, orthopedics, psychiatry, surgery, and urology, is commonly needed.

One widely discussed model of assessment service is the Department of Veteran Affairs (VA) geriatric evaluation unit. Rubenstein et al. (1984) evaluated the GEU at the Sepulveda VA Medical Center in Los Angeles. It was reported that after initial discharge, GEU patient rehospitalization was reduced (35 percent of GEU patients versus 50 percent of controls). Discharges to nursing homes were also reduced for GEU patients compared to control patients (13 percent versus 30 percent), as were the proportion of patients who were ever in a nursing home during the first year (27 percent versus 47 percent) and the average number of nursing home days (26 days versus 56 days). Total direct cost per year survived was reduced to $22,597, compared to $27,826 for control patients. The proportion of patients who improved in function sufficiently to be fully independent was increased (34 percent of GEU patients versus 29 percent of control patients). The jury is still out, however, on whether the heretofore unusually comprehensive nature of the geriatric assessment approach is cost-effective.

Outpatient Geriatric Assessment and Treatment. It would appear that focusing on near-acute patients with rehabilitation potential as a result of an initial physician-nurse-social worker assessment, and then augmenting this with a more comprehensive assessment and coordinated care program, might be a cost-effective way to introduce what appear to be some of the key (and most useful) features of geriatric assessment in our current Medicare fee-for-service system—at least for some types of near-acute care patients who do not require institutional care. In this regard, some geriatric assessment programs are using an outpatient rather than an inpatient approach in assessing and providing care to geriatric patients (Morishita et al. 1989; Williams et al. 1987; Hendriksen, Lund, and Stromgard 1989).

Morishita et al. (1989) describe an outpatient geriatric day hospital (GDH) based in a community hospital in Los Angeles, which is a hybrid of the VA's GEU, the British-model day hospital, and adult day health centers. This program is more expansive than that recommended above for consideration by Medicare. It could serve as the follow-up assessment program for patients judged to require a more comprehensive assessment. Geriatric care is provided on an outpatient basis in a hospital unit contiguous with a 12-bed inpatient geriatric ward. It consists of a day room (for socialization, meals, and group activities), a large area for physical and occupational therapy services, an exam room, a conference room, a nurses' station, and six patient rooms. All diagnostic and treatment services, except radiologic procedures, are performed in the day hospital itself. . . . Care is provided by an interdisciplinary team with expertise in geriatrics and gerontology. . . . Comprehensive geriatric assessment includes evaluation by the interdisciplinary team, completion of appropriate diagnostic tests, and consultations with medical specialists. The availability of acute nursing care enables patients who need hospital services such as blood transfusion to receive appropriate monitoring and treatment without overnight hospital stay. (Morishita et al. 1989, p. 337)

In general, the types of patients treated at the GDH were not as disabled as one typically encounters in GEUs. Thus, it appears that most GDH patients cannot be classified as near-acute care patients. Morishita et al. (1989) conducted a limited evaluation of the GDH based on interviews with 42 physicians who had referred patients to the GDH. They concluded that 21 percent of GDH patients had avoided a hospital admission, 7 percent were admitted for hospital care but with a shorter stay, 4 percent avoided nursing home admissions, and 44 percent substituted the GDH for other outpatient services.

A similar type of outpatient assessment intervention was operated by Monroe Community Hospital in Rochester, New York. Their Geriatric Ambulatory Consultative Service (GACS) provided outpatient assessment, treatment, and referral for clients whose functional status was about the same as patients eligible for intermediate-level nursing home care in New York State. In a randomized, controlled evaluation (Williams et al. 1987), hospital admissions were reported to be unchanged, but length of stay was reduced 39 percent for the GACS patients. Thus, the increased cost of assessment services ($350) was more than offset by reductions in the use of other health care services. Relative to total costs for control clients, the program was reported to have produced a net saving of 25 percent ($2,189) per client. For the most part, it appears that outpatient geriatric assessment units concentrate on patients with more chronic or maintenance care needs. They are therefore less relevant to our objectives here, which focus on near-acute care largely for patients with rehabilitation potential. Nonetheless, their experience suggests that it may be possible to provide certain types of near-acute care using an outpatient approach to geriatric assessment and treatment.

Geriatric Assessment and Near-Acute Care. Kane, Kane, and Rubenstein (1989) reviewed 31 studies of comprehensive functional assessment of the elderly within the context of health care. As a result of this review, they reported that the structure of assessment interventions varies widely and that outcomes are not readily comparable between studies. They reported that the preponderance of evidence indicates that systematic assessment of the elderly is of significant value. Nevertheless, the authors cautioned that this is an expensive, labor-intensive service that should be carefully targeted toward "those at greatest risk and those most likely to benefit from the proposed intervention" (Kane, Kane, and Rubenstein 1989, p. 509).

The number of proponents of GEUs and GACs is growing in the health care field. The more committed proponents contend there is really no need to even evaluate the effectiveness of such programs empirically (although evaluations are underway, with early evidence arguably suggesting that the programs are effective). Some advocates say the approach is so characterized by common sense and the dictates of good health care that we should not bother evaluating its effectiveness. Rather, we should simply do it (Eubanks 1989). They readily admit it will cost more to do the assessment correctly at the outset of a near-acute care stay but contend it will more than pay for itself in terms of improved quality of life, reduced subsequent hospitalization, avoidance of chronic institutional long-term care, and improved patient health status that lessens the need for health services in general.

Others do not embrace it, however, contending that it has not been thoroughly evaluated (Cohen and Feussner 1989) or that it may be too complex, cumbersome, and costly to do on a widespread basis (Bernstein 1989). At this writing, the VA is in the process of designing two multistate trials to more comprehensively test the cost effectiveness of the GEU approach. In formulating a national policy for near-acute care, a more measured approach would dictate that we isolate the essential features, thereby minimizing its cost, while initially targeting patient conditions for which geriatric assessment is most likely to be cost-effective.

Ongoing Programs, Provider Experimentation, and Research

The Sudden Decline Experiment. An inpatient program designed to provide near-acute and even acute care in skilled nursing facilities was described by Zimmer et al. (1988). Termed the "sudden decline" benefit, the intent of the program was to avoid hospitalizing nursing home patients who experience a sudden decline in health status that might typically warrant an episode of hospital care. It combined increased availability of physician services in nursing homes with a somewhat more generous nursing home reimbursement rate in order to prevent both hospital inpatient care and emergency care.

The benefit is administered as follows. When the nursing home staff determines that a patient is suffering from an acute problem, the physician is notified immediately. [The program] pays both the nursing home to complete a comprehensive patient assessment and a physician to examine and treat the patient in a nursing home. Associated diagnostic tests and procedures are also reimbursed. . . . If the patient remains in the nursing home, the nursing home can authorize up to 14 days of payments. . . . The physician is paid to visit daily as long as the patient is medically eligible for the . . . benefit, up to 100 days. (Zimmer et al. 1988, p. 125)

Employing an independent three-member committee of physicians to review the medical records of the first 112 patients in the program, an assessment of the likelihood of hospitalization was made for each patient under the assumption that the sudden decline program would not have been available to the patient. The physician assessment committee concluded that 76 percent of the patients were saved either inpatient hospitalization or an emergency room visit. The predominant services provided consisted of physician examination (all cases), skilled nursing observation (all cases), chest x-rays (42 cases), blood tests (36 cases), intake and output measurement (27 cases), parenteral therapy (25 cases), oxygen therapy (20 cases), suctioning and tracheostomy acute care (12 cases), and nasogastric tube (11 cases).

In all, the authors reached the conclusion that considerable savings accrued to both Medicare and Medicaid as a result of the program. The study estimated that the cost saving to Medicare was over $3,000 per patient. The authors concluded that "the financial coverage of daily physician visits to the SNF is essential to the success of this approach, as is the assurance that the necessary intensive acute nursing, and other services can be provided adequately in SNFs. . . . The potential for cost saving is considerable" (Zimmer et al. 1988, p. 125).

New Programs and Philosophies in Near-Acute and Transitional Care. As the number of hard-to-place patients discharged from hospitals continues to increase, various larger hospitals in metropolitan areas have begun to experiment with different approaches to postdischarge planning and care. It is now apparent in many locations that the hospital discharge plan is either inadequate or, in cases where it is adequate, is simply not followed. Hospital discharge planners are not always inclined to follow up to determine whether such plans are implemented, since there are often few financial incentives to do so. John Selsted of the Ebenezer Society Center for Aging in Minnesota states, "The cutting edge is to coordinate the physician, the hospital, the nursing home, home health care, and family caregivers. When providers respond with new models of collaboration and coordination, the whole system benefits" (Beresford 1990, p. 2).

The phrase "short-term long-term care" (STLTC), a term that appears to have been first coined by Eileen Tynan in the 1970s for swing-bed care provided in Texas, Iowa, and South Dakota, has recently been resurrected in a manner synonymous with near-acute care. For example, Stanley Brody refers to STLTC as "near-term rehabilitation to improve elderly patients' functioning" and is distinct from "traditional long-term custodial care for patients who will require the current level of services for the rest of their lives" (Beresford 1990). Programs in various hospitals in the Twin Cities, including Hennepin County Medical Center and Ramsey County Hospital in St. Paul, have undertaken a coordinated approach to acute care and long-term care by assigning various health professionals, including physicians, to continue following patient progress through telephone or in-person visits after discharge. While reimbursement is typically not available for such activities, they are encouraged to lessen rehospitalizations for either uninsured or underinsured patients (Beresford 1990).

The Robert Wood Johnson Foundation (RWJF) has a program entitled "Hospital Initiatives in Long-Term Care," under which it has awarded grants to 24 hospital systems for purposes of encouraging systemwide care coordination and case management. The approach is premised on the fact that hospitals represent key entry points into the long-term care system and, in general, our health care system.

Another RWJF initiative that promotes integrated near-acute care has been implemented at the Albany Medical Center Hospital in New York State. It has several of the characteristics of an outpatient day hospital since the program is intended to provide more intensive transitional daytime care to patients at high risk of complications, including hospital readmissions. The intent of the program is to improve health outcomes and lower the cost of care for such patients.

Many of these types of programs have a major drawback from the perspective of third party payers, including Medicare: The idea of coordinated care or, to use an older phrase, case management typically implies a second type of care that payers have not traditionally covered. This management or monitoring function can be done in a variety of ways. In the original "channeling" demonstrations, this role was often played by an independent individual such as a person with a social services background, termed the *case manager*. There now exist certain follow-up programs that simply provide follow-up data collection and monitoring services for purposes of either quality assurance or case management. In any event, payers tend to resist covering such services because these individuals are not direct providers of health or medical care—and are viewed as increasing the short-run cost of such care. However, evidence is now available strongly suggesting that such services, when properly structured and targeted, can actually lower long-run cost, particularly for near-acute care patients.

Geriatric Nurse Clinicians and Geriatric Nurse Practitioners. Mathy Mezey uses the phrase "geriatric nurse clinicians" to describe individuals who are master's- or doctoral-prepared nurses with an emphasis in geriatric or gerontological care. Such individuals were among the mainstays of the teaching nursing home program (TNHP) that she administered for the Robert Wood Johnson Foundation. As mentioned, the program was successful in reducing hospitalizations for nursing home patients. Geriatric nurse clinicians were involved in comprehensive assessments of patient care needs, while working with and training nurses aides as well as other nursing staff in nursing homes that were formally affiliated with schools of nursing in several sites throughout the United States.

The involvement of geriatric nurse clinicians in long-term care was evaluated in the TNHP (Shaughnessy, Kramer, and Hittle 1990). The precise extent to which it could be used in other nursing homes or transported more systematically to near-acute care settings is unknown. Yet it bears considerable promise, since the TNHP evaluation provided evidence suggesting that geriatric nurse clinicians can enhance the quality of long-term care in nursing homes or nursing home–like environments.

The TNHP geriatric nurse clinician model has certain attributes similar to the swing-bed approach used in rural hospitals in providing long-term care. In swing-bed hospitals, the directors of nursing, charge nurses, and at times swing-bed coordinators, in instances where they were members of the nursing staff, were typically nurses more experienced and well-trained in acute care and, by extension, many aspects of near-acute long-term care. Nursing staff under their supervision, including other registered nurses, licensed practical nurses, and aides and orderlies, often received more instruction and direct supervision in various aspects of near-acute care (such as attentiveness to specific types of signs and symptoms, and monitoring vital signs consistently) than is typically the case in most nursing homes. The lower rehospitalization rates for near-acute care patients treated in swing-bed hospitals were a manifestation of this. Diligence in encouraging patient independence and rehabilitation also characterized geriatric nurse clinician care in the TNHP and the more therapeutic approach to skilled nursing in swing-bed hospitals. Just as with the parallel between GEUs and the swing-bed approach in comprehensively assessing patient care needs, the swing-bed approach was not as formalized in its use of nursing staff as was the TNHP in its use of geriatric nurse clinicians. It simply evolved naturally and persists today, but could perhaps benefit further from a more systematic and rigorous specification of activities involved.

Unlike geriatric nurse clinicians, geriatric nurse practitioners are not necessarily master's-trained. They may, in fact, be nonbachelor's-prepared nurses with an educational certificate from a geriatric nurse practitioner program. Two demonstration programs, one in the mountain states and the other in Massachusetts, were conducted and evaluated during the early 1980s (Kane, Garrard, Buchanan, et al. 1989; Kane, Garrard, Skay, et al. 1989; Kane, Kane, et al. 1988; Buchanan et al. 1989; Master et al. 1980). The presence of geriatric nurse practitioners in nursing homes appeared to reduce hospitalization rates, although it did not appear to have any other significant effects on quality of care that could explain the reasons for the decreases in hospitalization (Garrard et al. 1990). Administrators and directors of nursing, however, expressed greater satisfaction with the nurse practitioner approach than the traditional approach (Buchanan et al. 1989). In general, the geriatric nurse practitioner programs did not impose as pervasive a change as did the teaching nursing home approach. Nevertheless, they emphasized better assessment and integration of long-term care in nursing homes. As a result, they constitute a step in the direction not only of more comprehensive geriatric assessment, but also, in the case of the Massachusetts program especially, a closer integration with physician care.

Opportunities for Managed Care Innovations. Health maintenance organizations (HMOs) represent a potential natural experimental setting for examining better coordinated acute, long-term, and ambulatory care. This is not to say that such care is in fact better coordinated in HMOs, since the anecdotal evidence available is far from definitive. Yet, it would appear that some HMOs are undertaking rather innovative care programs that should facilitate a better coordinated approach to long-term care than we might have in our fee-for-service system. It would also appear, however, that these HMOs are the exception rather than the rule, since a large number of HMOs contract to outside providers for long-term care services, often seeking to minimize the utilization of such services to control costs, somewhat independently of whether the services might be effective, cost-effective, or in the best interest of patients.

Nonetheless, the subjective evidence available on selected HMOs that own and operate home health agencies as part of their total program suggests that home health care is being used in a more widespread and aggressive manner, often combined with outpatient and ambulatory care, for near-acute care patients—with a view toward avoiding hospitalization and enhancing rehabilitation. This also appears to be the case for SNF care in a few HMO settings that own or lease SNF beds. Such beds are at times used for near-acute care patients with rehabilitation potential in order to avoid hospital care and maximize functional outcomes. At times, such HMOs have extended care coordinators and geriatricians who are medical directors or part-time medical directors in their long-term care facilities.

It is to be emphasized, however, that HMOs are not being advocated here as models of coordinated long-term care. There is no evidence to suggest that the above-mentioned innovations are occurring except in unusual cases. In fact, some feel that a number of HMOs are further behind in terms of well-coordinated long-term care than our fee-for-service system. Regardless, the main point here is that at least selected HMO programs would appear to warrant further study from the viewpoint of well-coordinated long-term care programs, especially programs that involve near-acute care patients.

Expanding and Contracting Medicare SNF Care under the Catastrophic Coverage Act

The Medicare Catastrophic Coverage Act (MCCA) of 1988 (P.L. 100-360) changed the Medicare SNF benefit considerably until its repeal approximately 18 months after its enactment. The Medicare SNF benefit was changed largely by increasing the number of Medicare-covered SNF days from 100 to 150 per year, substantially decreasing the coinsurance that the Medicare beneficiary had to pay, and eliminating the requirement that a Medicare SNF patient be discharged from a hospital within 30 days prior to an SNF admission. Critics of this liberalization of the Medicare SNF benefit under the MCCA contended that it opened the floodgates for a radical increase in Medicare expenditures on SNF care. Total SNF costs under the Medicare program tripled in one year's time during the period when the provisions of the MCCA were in effect, from $99 million/month in 1988 to $300 million in June of 1989 (Migdail 1989). Nevertheless, the primary reason for this increase in Medicare SNF expenditures is presently unclear, since clarifications to the coverage guidelines for Medicare SNF care went into effect at about the same time.

In effect, under MCCA, Medicare had ventured into the traditional long-term care business for the first time in history. The expanded SNF benefit resulted in Medicare underwriting Medicaid expenses for some nursing home patients. The previous Medicare SNF reimbursement policies were much more stringent, not only requiring a three-day prior hospital stay, but also requiring greater copayment by the patient and restricting the number of days that Medicare would cover SNF care. For many types of patients, the differences between the expanded Medicare SNF coverage under the Catastrophic Coverage Act and earlier Medicare SNF coverage policies were previously covered by Medicaid. Some states were left in a lurch with the repeal of this aspect of the Catastrophic Coverage Act in late 1989 since they had developed their new Medicaid budgets under the assumption that certain nursing home costs would be covered by Medicare.

This Medicare foray into the traditional long-term care field was brief and rather unpleasant for policymakers and many concerned about nursing home coverage. Paraphrasing the reaction of proponents of Medicare's approach to long-term care, "From the viewpoint of institutional care, Medicare is basically in the acute care business, not the traditional long-term care business which is the domain of Medicaid. The ECF under Medicare was intended to provide some degree of near-acute care with the intent of lowering the cost of care toward the end of an otherwise too lengthy hospital stay and avoiding rehospitalizations for certain types of patients." In all likelihood, for better or for worse, repeal of the Catastrophic Coverage Act more firmly ensconced this historic acute care Medicare orientation in the eyes of many policymakers. To quote a congressional staffer, "It will be a long time before we substantially expand the Medicare long-term care benefit again." If one looks at the ebb and flow of Medicare reimbursement policy over the last two and one-half decades, however, it may not be very long. Perhaps sometime during the 1990s, we may once again see this benefit altered because of the rapidly changing needs for long-term care in this country. Such a forecast will not necessarily help us in the short run, however, when we are confronted with a fragmented and, at best, patchwork approach to providing near-acute care.

WHERE IS SWING-BED CARE GOING?

Swing Beds in Larger Rural Hospitals

Section 405(b) of the Omnibus Budget Reconciliation Act of 1987 (P.L. 100-203) expanded the original swing-bed program under Section 904 of OBRA 1980 (P.L. 96-499) by extending the swing-bed program to rural hospitals with less than 100 beds. The expansion of the bed size limit from 49 to 99 included additional restrictions for larger hospitals that would participate under this new and second version of the swing-bed program, while the first version remained intact with fewer restrictions for hospitals with less than 50 beds (Grim 1990). The regulations for the second rural swing-bed program for larger hospitals were published on September 7, 1989 (HCFA 1989b).

The new program required swing-bed hospitals to transfer Medicare SNF patients to Medicare SNFs within five days unless a physician certifies otherwise; to have transfer and availability agreements with SNFs for purposes of transferring swing-bed patients to such facilities in their communities; and not to provide an excessive amount of swing-bed care—where excessive is defined to be more than 15 percent of all acute care beds occupied by long-term care patients over a 12-month period. While the original swing-bed legislation and regulations corresponding to Section 904 of OBRA 1980 encouraged smaller swing-bed hospitals to transfer patients to SNFs, the requirements were by no means as stringent as those required under OBRA 1987. Section 4008(j) of OBRA 1990 (P.L. 101-508) further amended the national program by setting Medicare (routine cost) payments to swing-bed hospitals to the same level as payments to freestanding Medicare SNFs. Provision was made, however, for hospitals that exceed this limit to be reimbursed at the prior rate until such time that the new limit exceeds current payment. This section of OBRA 1990 also allowed hospitals that had entered the program prior to May 1, 1987 to remain in the program regardless of whether the area in which they are located is no longer considered rural. The fact that OBRA 1990 in effect increased reimbursement for many swing-bed hospitals by raising payments to those received by freestanding Medicare SNFs has made the swing-bed approach more attractive to eligible hospitals.

Therefore, it is more advantageous for a hospital to qualify under the original swing-bed program for smaller hospitals than under the second swing-bed program for larger hospitals. It is, in fact, likely that a number of hospitals seeking to enter the swing-bed program will have their choice since, even for larger hospitals, bed size is determined by the number of staffed beds. Thus, if an 80-bed hospital only staffs and uses 45 of its beds, it is eligible under the original swing-bed program. The exact manner in which growth will continue under the original program relative to the second, more restrictive program for larger hospitals remains to be seen. Nonetheless, the second program clearly highlights an emphasis on short-term near-acute care, although it continues to restrict swing beds to rural hospitals.

Mandated restrictions that require use of an empty SNF bed and the five-day limit, however, are very likely excessive and represent a capitulation to concerns of the nursing home industry. By early 1991, relatively few rural hospitals with 50–99 beds had joined the swing-bed program under the OBRA 1987 provision. Paraphrasing a nursing home administrator who was supporting an unsuccessful attempt to repeal the original swing-bed program in a midwestern state, "These swing-bed hospitals are now beginning to cut into my business. After discharging an acute care patient, they care for them in their own swing beds for another two to three weeks, rehabilitating them so they can be discharged home. I'm losing business because I never see them in my facility. Some of these patients are the types that would have stayed for years in my nursing home. Something has to be done about this swing-bed program."

As mentioned, opposition from the nursing home industry was minimal throughout the 1970s and during the first half of the 1980s (North Dakota State Health Council 1989). It appears, however, that nursing home occupancy rates may have dropped in certain rural swing-bed communities in the latter part of the 1980s, probably due to some combination of three factors in the communities where it is occurring. First, the populations in a number of rural communities are decreasing in size, including the elderly (i.e., counter to the trend of an increasing elderly population nationally). Second, the rehabilitation care to which the above administrator was referring is unusually effective for several types of patients, thereby laudably reducing the demand for traditional long-term care services for such patients. Third, in some communities, swing-bed hospitals are competing more directly with nursing homes for traditional long-term care patients. As noted earlier, this third phenomenon tends to remain the exception rather than the rule in view of the extremely short stays for swing-bed patients relative to nursing home patients. Such care does not cost payers any more than nursing home care, however, and some patients prefer a swing-bed hospital setting to a nursing home setting (in those relatively few instances where swing-bed hospitals undertake the provision of traditional long-term care). We must also ask ourselves whether a modicum of competition (which is all that could be possibly offered in the traditional long-term care field by the swing-bed program) is good or bad. Regardless, the empirical evidence that has been accumulated to date suggests that wholesale provision of traditional long-term care in swing-bed hospitals is something to be avoided. In view of the diminutive number of long-stay swing-bed patients, this possibility remains far from a reality and certainly does not appear to be something we should legislate against.

Continued Growth and Potential Expansion of the Swing-Bed Approach

Since the various policy initiatives described at the outset of this chapter (e.g., deinstitutionalization, Medicaid preadmission screening, a proliferation of home- and community-based care programs, and PPS) have had a substantial impact on the demand for near-acute care services, we are confronted with the dual question of whether and how to satisfy this demand. A hard-line response to this question is premised on the assumption that a sufficient cushion was built into hospital care and reimbursement under Medicare by the early 1980s, and that near-acute care was really covered under the DRG rates initially established; therefore, hospitals should be able to provide such care at the end of an acute stay without additional reimbursement to either hospital-based or freestanding providers of near-acute care. Others would argue that either such a cushion was not built into the initial DRG rates, or that they have been racheted down so tightly over the years that now reimbursement is inadequate to cover the cost of near-acute care through DRG rates for hospitals. At this stage, the latter argument appears to have cogency, particularly in view of the potential gains that can be reaped from properly providing near-acute care, including gains in both cost and quality of care.

Because the rural swing-bed program was unusually successful in providing at least certain types of near-acute care, the temptation to expand it almost unilaterally to urban and larger hospitals is strong. Yet common sense would dictate that caution should be exercised. First, the multiplicity of health care providers and alternatives for providing long-term care that characterize urban communities paints a considerably different picture from the limited and often nonexistent options that characterize many rural communities.

Second, evidence currently available suggests that some urban communities are confronted with strong unmet demand for near-acute care services and have relatively few certified nursing homes able to admit patients with complex near-acute care needs, while other communities seem to have minimal problems at best in this regard. We simply do not know enough about the reasons for this considerable variation across metropolitan areas.

Third, introducing a swing-bed approach in urban hospitals perforce raises several questions that were not necessarily applicable to rural hospitals. For example, how many beds and what types of beds can and should be swung in a 500-bed tertiary care facility? Should stronger precautionary steps be taken to ensure that abuses of the swing-bed approach do not occur in larger hospitals? The more sophisticated financial capabilities and potential to maximize reimbursement increase the likelihood of such abuse. Why bother with a swing-bed approach in urban hospitals where large numbers of beds often go unoccupied in this post-PPS era? There is quite a difference between a small rural 40-bed hospital, where a 50 percent occupancy rate leaves but 20 empty beds, and a 400-bed hospital, where it leaves 200 empty beds. If we have a demand for near-acute services, should we not simply convert a certain number of hospital beds to hospital-based SNF beds, thereby ignoring the swing-bed approach altogether?

Since the secretary of Health and Human Services still has demonstration authority for a swing-bed approach under Section 904 of OBRA 1980, would it not be wise to try some sort of a demonstration in this regard, rather than implement a swing-bed approach on a widespread basis? We must ask whether the most attractive feature of the swing-bed approach focuses on the practice of swinging a hospital bed between acute and long-term care, or whether there is another attribute that really is the defining characteristic of this successful program in rural communities? Is it not the fact that we have discovered a rather rudimentary way to provide near-acute care, which, with some degree of refinement, we can reshape to meet the rapidly growing near-acute care needs of our elderly population in a far more cost-effective way than we are presently doing? In fact, we are now at the point where the swing-bed concept should be subservient to this goal, to the point of downplaying the term *swing-bed care* substituting *near-acute care* in its place, and moving forward with how to best provide such care. This issue is addressed in the next chapter.

POLICY CONSIDERATIONS RELEVANT TO NEAR-ACUTE CARE

What We Are Integrating

If one were to plot the combined nursing, medical, and technological care needs of long-term care on a continuum according to levels of provider skill and training required, traditional long-term care patients would tend to be at the low to mid-range of this continuum, while near-acute care patients would be at the high end of the continuum. Note the continuum under discussion focuses on professional skills, training, and expertise—not cost, resource consumption, morbidity, risk of mortality, or even perceived importance of care. In fact, it has been validly argued that sometimes chronic care or traditional long-term care patients with substantial functional, emotional, and/or cognitive needs can be as costly to care for as near-acute patients (Vladeck 1987b). In this regard, there is probably not a valid continuum of care with respect to resource consumption or cost (or morbidity, mortality risk, or importance of care), although there appears to be such a continuum with respect to training needed to acquire needed skill levels on the part of care providers. The continuum of provider skills under consideration includes more than functional care (needs for such care are often of paramount importance and may be strongest for traditional or chronic long-term care patients); near-acute care patients may or may not be functionally impaired. What distinguishes near-acute patients from traditional long-term care patients is their intensified needs for services that are at times found in acute care settings, such as diagnostic services, increased physician care, physical or rehabilitation therapy, more frequent monitoring of medical problems, IV medications, ventilator care, postsurgical care, and a variety of skilled nursing services provided by RNs.

A number of providers are currently involved in near-acute care. Not only do certain types of nursing homes and swing-bed hospitals provide such care, but a reasonable amount of such care is presently provided in acute care hospital beds without reimbursement or through provisions for the administratively necessary days provision under the Medicaid programs in some states. Various states permit such care to be provided in acute care hospital beds when no nursing home beds are available. On the other hand, these types of payment arrangements for hospitals are usually considered to be temporary and undesirable from the viewpoint of the payers.

PPS-exempt rehabilitation hospitals provide near-acute care to selected types of patients, especially those who require substantial amounts of therapy. For a patient to be classified as an inpatient in a Medicare rehabilitation hospital, he or she must be able to undergo an extensive amount of rehabilitation care on a daily basis; for example, the patient must require at least three hours of physical or occupational therapy daily. Regulations also call for 24-hour availability of physicians and nurses with specialized training in rehabilitation, frequent physician involvement, and a program of care coordinated by a multidisciplinary team (Gornick and Hall 1988). Owing to the unusually intensive care required by and provided to such patients, this type of facility (i.e., a PPS-exempt rehabilitation hospital) is typically as costly as an acute care hospital—more so at times. In theory, such facilities treat patients that are therefore acute care patients in terms of the intensity of their care needs, but who do not receive typical inpatient hospital care. The rehabilitation programs and regimens at such facilities are of a different nature and intensity than is the case for near-acute care as discussed here. It is entirely possible, however, that some patients are inappropriately classified as rehabilitation hospital patients and might be candidates for the types of near-acute care alternatives discussed in this book. As Medicare officials continue to examine eligibility and reimbursement policy for PPS-exempt rehabilitation hospitals, relationships with near-acute care cases and providers of near-acute care should be taken into consideration.

Some hospitals use the term *transitional care unit* to refer to a PPS-exempt rehabilitation hospital that is part of an extant acute care hospital. Such units were set up in the mid- and late 1980s in various hospitals throughout the country and, in certain instances, in freestanding facilities specializing in rehabilitation that may have existed prior to PPS. These units provide intense rehabilitation care for hard-to-place patients who have such intense service needs that the staff of many Medicare SNFs prefer not to admit them. In other settings and in other locations, however, the term *transitional care* is used more broadly, as discussed above.

Some near-acute care is provided by Medicare-certified home health agencies. The substantial increase in Medicare-certified home health care during the 1980s was accompanied by an increase in high-tech home health care. In order to provide the variety of near-acute care services that are often necessary for a given patient, we must somehow integrate services that are commonly found in inpatient hospital settings, nursing home settings, and even outpatient and in-home settings. Health care professionals, such as physicians, skilled nurses, physical therapists, social workers, and even home health practitioners, have to coordinate the provision of services and exchange of patient information. Monitoring patient status relative to expected goals and prognoses that were initially established in one setting, but require follow-up in other settings, is frequently essential. Right now our basic fee-for-service payment system, under which each provider tends to bill for and be reimbursed separately for the services he or she provides, leads not only to fragmentation in reimbursement, but also more importantly, fragmentation in patient care with potential inefficiencies and inadequate communication resulting in poor or substandard patient outcomes.

Flexible Regulations

It is easy to state that we should have a flexible regulatory system. Very few would disagree with this on the basis of general principles. On the other hand, a clear and evenhanded approach to specifying and enforcing regulations is difficult. When a law is passed or a general policy is made in health care, regulations are typically necessary to clarify the exact nature of program administration, associated rules, and the manner in which the rules should be followed. It is appropriate that exceptions to regulatory standards be relatively few. Regulatory agencies have difficulty enforcing standards that require significant individual judgment on whether a provider is either in or out of compliance. Further, difficulties are posed when such agencies have to "semienforce" the standards. For example, the swing-bed approach was implemented with the condition that certain regulatory standards that apply to nursing

homes should not apply to swing-bed hospitals. The spirit of the regulations was such that agencies should be a bit more lenient with swing-
bed hospitals than nursing homes.

Yet this is what is required under certain circumstances where
long-term care innovations are under consideration. We must be able to
have some degree of flexibility in our regulatory system so that we
neither overregulate nor seriously impede innovation and improvement
in our delivery system. In this regard, regulators, researchers, and policy analysts must function together so that we might satisfy the spirit as
well as the letter of regulatory objectives that are designed to foster
innovation. At times, this can best be accomplished through demonstration projects.

Using Empty Hospital Beds

Most people agree we have too many hospital beds in the United States.
The issue of what to do about it is far from straightforward, however.
Since hospital occupancy rates have fallen substantially over the last
decade, largely due to incentives for early discharge resulting from PPS,
it is apparent that some beds should be closed. The cost of maintaining
"mothballed" hospital beds may not be as substantial as some originally
feared (Pauly and Wilson 1986), but disagreement still exists on just how
much it costs to maintain an empty hospital bed (Mickel 1989). Regardless, it is a fact that wholesale closures of hospital beds simply have not
occurred to the degree some had forecast, although a reasonable number of hospital beds are no longer staffed or maintained for hospital care.
Such closures serve to reduce institutional costs to some extent, in keeping with the original intent of regulators and formulators of changes in
reimbursement policy designed to control increases in hospital costs.

If a given hospital staffs and maintains beds for acute care under
the presumption that a certain volume of such care is needed by the
community it serves, it makes sense to consider uses of such beds when
they are not occupied by acute care patients. The swing-bed approach
has been premised on this assumption and proven successful in minimizing cost. The question has been asked, Why not convert acute care
beds to nursing home beds or long-term care beds instead of bothering
with the swing-bed program? First, this has been done in many instances. However, the swing-bed program is premised on the assumption that staffed but empty hospital beds may be necessary for acute care
and should be used when possible. It is also premised on the assumption that there is an unmet need in the community for relatively small
amounts of near-acute care that cannot be effectively satisfied by providers with limited access to acute care services. (In this regard, a "small
amount" is a function of hospital size.) As shown in Chapters 5 and 6, a

small amount of long-term care can be provided more cost-effectively in acute care beds used as swing beds than it can by converting acute care beds to long-term care beds.

As also noted in Chapter 6 a break-even or threshold point exists for each hospital. This threshold point, expressed as a given number of swing-bed days for a particular hospital, is where the cost of swing-bed care exceeds revenues when the hospital provides an amount of swing-bed care in excess of the threshold. The threshold point is reached when it is necessary to staff a certain number of additional beds for long-term care that were not already staffed for acute care. If a hospital attains an average daily census of swing-bed patients that is greater than this threshold value, it then makes sense from the hospital's perspective to convert its swing beds to long-term care beds since Medicare SNF reimbursement would be more generous than swing-bed reimbursement under the existing national program. Further, an average daily census that is sufficiently high connotes that the hospital is in the long-term care business, functioning as a nursing home, and very likely specializing in near-acute care in this instance. Therefore, the beds should be configured structurally as nursing home beds, and the appropriate staff mix and other regulatory requirements for nursing homes should be satisfied.

It makes sense, however, for this to be a hospital-level decision, since third party payers such as Medicare and Medicaid actually pay less for swing-bed care than for nursing home care. Market forces would naturally dictate bed conversion decisions of this nature in a hospital setting, without the need for regulatory intervention. However, if a swing-bed hospital were providing large amounts of chronic long-term care in such beds (i.e., to long-stay patients), it might be appropriate to treat such a facility as a nursing home from a regulatory perspective. This would be in keeping with the finding that swing-bed hospitals, although unusually successful in providing near-acute care, do not provide chronic long-term care as effectively as nursing homes. Only if the hospital is providing an extensive amount of chronic long-term care without converting swing beds to nursing home beds should intervention occur. Since this has rarely occurred to date, it is not perceived to be a problem that warrants extensive regulatory scrutiny. It could be easily monitored by assessing total days of care and average length of stay (which is considerably longer for typical chronic care patients than for near-acute care patients).

SNF Reimbursement and Administratively Necessary Days

Reimbursement for Medicare SNFs is cost-based up to limits that are different for freestanding and hospital-based nursing homes. Further,

Medicare SNFs that provide fewer than 1,500 days of Medicare-covered care are free to choose whether they wish to be paid in this manner or on the basis of a prospectively determined flat rate set at 105 percent of the mean operating and capital costs of all Medicare SNFs. As case mix has intensified during the 1980s, reluctance to admit certain types of near-acute patients to Medicare SNFs has increased. According to many in the nursing home industry at least, Medicare reimbursement is not adequate to cover the resource requirements of such patients. Hard-to-place Medicare SNF patients therefore often remain in acute care beds (in non-swing-bed hospitals) after discharge from acute care. These extra days in acute care hospitals are often referred to as administratively necessary days (ANDs). Holahan et al. (1989) defined ANDs as days "when a patient remains in the hospital because of inability to place the patient in a nursing home." In fact, the AND problem dates back to well before PPS. Medicare typically does not pay for such days, although a provision in Section 902 of the Omnibus Budget Reconciliation Act of 1980 (P.L. 96-499) allows for Medicare reimbursement for administratively necessary days. This particular option has rarely, if ever, been exercised.

Nevertheless, the backlog of postacute patients in hospitals is a serious problem in some areas such as New York State. In some states, the state Medicaid program has payment policies that cover ANDs for Medicaid-eligible patients. Holahan et al. (1989) point out that hospitals with their own SNF unit (hospital-based Medicare-certified nursing homes) or swing beds are able to discharge patients more quickly than hospitals with no control over nursing home beds. Consequently, such hospitals would appear to be at a financial advantage under PPS. As pointed out in Chapters 5 and 6, swing-bed hospitals nonetheless function cost-effectively by virtue of enhanced patient outcomes and lower total cost to Medicare. In all, it would appear that, properly structured, incentives for increased physician care and increased involvement of qualified institutional providers of near-acute care can result in higher-quality care and lower cost to society. It appears that by targeting SNF patients (perhaps circumscribing particular types of near-acute care patients, such as those with rehabilitation potential) who need more intense SNF services, we could take a strong step in the direction of better integrating acute care and long-term care.

An issue that has been under consideration by both Medicare officials and the Office of Management and Budget is bundling acute care with SNF services under a single reimbursement mechanism; for example, serious consideration was recently given to bundling hospital care and postacute SNF or home health care reimbursement under a single DRG payment. For the approach under consideration, hospitals would have been responsible for directly providing or subcontracting posthospital care in return for a certain percentage increase in their DRG rates. This was opposed by a number of provider and even governmental representatives. From a substantive perspective, it would appear premature to bundle hospital and SNF services in this manner since there is so little known about the direct relationship between acute care and long-term care as a function of acute care patient characteristics alone. In fact, many in the long-term care field argue validly that acute care diagnoses alone are relatively unimportant as determinants of resource needs for postacute long-term care. The very fact that such bundling was given a reasonable degree of consideration, however, points to the recognition that enhanced coordination of acute and near-acute services has appeal from the perspective of cost effectiveness.

Physician Reimbursement

Within the medical field, geriatrics is a rapidly evolving field, as evidenced by these quotes.

> Geriatrics faces a special challenge. Geriatricians aim to preserve or restore functional ability despite many chronic conditions, to support the older person's ability to cope with inevitable physical and emotional changes, to establish reasonable therapeutic goals, and to minimize the risk of iatrogenic complications by limiting medications and procedures to those that are absolutely essential. This work requires time, skill, and patience, and generally avoids invasive, expensive procedures. (Butler and Hyer 1989, p. 1,097)

> Geriatrics is the clinical care of a particular group of older persons. Nearly all patients in a geriatric practice are Medicare beneficiaries, though most Medicare beneficiaries are not geriatric patients. The orientation of geriatrics is to "a group of people defined not simply by age, but representing a complex syndrome of multiple, simultaneous, interactive problems that necessitate a functional approach to the patient, with a strong emphasis on comprehensive assessment." [Kane 1988a, p. 468] The interacting problems are not only medical but also economic, psychological, and social. . . . The geriatric approach to the patient "is more comprehensive, looking at the totality of the patient and focusing on the patient rather than simply on diseases or syndromes . . . working with both the medical and social components of the patient's problems" [Kane 1988a, p. 468]. (Hammons and Pawlson 1989, p. 1,085)

> Medicare reimbursement policy may have a greater effect on geriatric practice than on other specialties. Geriatrics is the only specialty that is exclusively focused on the care of Medicare patients and, in addition, oriented to Medicare beneficiaries with complex medical and psychosocial problems. If Medicare provides inadequate reimbursement for a given visit, the costs cannot be shifted to patients with other insurance coverage. Recognizing the heavy illness burden, high medical expenses, and limited income of many of the so-called frail elderly, many geriatricians may be

> reluctant to refuse assignment and balance-bill. . . . The adoption of a resource-based fee schedule would increase the payment for most geriatric services. (Hammons and Pawlson 1989, p. 1,090)

This recommendation, made both by Hammons and Pawlson, and by Butler and Hyer (1989), was directed to the Physician Payment Review Commission (PPRC), responsible for a resource-based fee schedule with limits on balance billing as the primary mechanism for Medicare payment for physician services.

Since several studies have shown that increased physician involvement in the near-acute care field is cost-effective, it would appear that this is an area that warrants very serious consideration. Specifically, reimbursement for more physician visits and physician involvement in assessment of near-acute patients is likely to benefit patients and payers alike through decreased hospital use by near-acute care patients. This would also provide a step in the direction of greater recognition of the immense potential of the field of geriatrics for elderly Americans.

The Roles of Medicare and Medicaid in Long-Term Care

Although the Catastrophic Coverage Act of 1988 (P.L. 100-360) brought about a small but temporary change, Medicare as a public payer has never entered the traditional public payer domain of Medicaid in the long-term care field. Medicaid pays for about 40 percent of all nursing home care in the United States (HCFA 1987). Roughly 40 percent of each Medicaid dollar in a typical state also goes to nursing home care (HCFA 1989c). While there are some exceptions to this (i.e., considerably higher proportions in some states and lower proportions in others go to nursing home care), Medicaid is in the nursing home business in a big way throughout the country. By contrast, less than 2 percent of Medicare Part A expenditures are spent on SNF care (HCFA 1989c). Under the swing-bed program, this was reversed. Since swing-bed hospitals emphasize near-acute care, Medicare pays for approximately 50 percent of all swing-bed days in the United States; Medicaid pays for only about 8 percent, partly because it does not even participate as a payer for swing-bed care in many states.

We discussed earlier how swing-bed care is saving Medicare money by decreasing acute care for SNF patients through its participation in the swing-bed program. The swing-bed program is most likely saving state Medicaid programs money on nursing home care by virtue of higher community discharge rates for patients who might have been otherwise admitted to nursing homes. Many state Medicaid programs have been reluctant to participate in the swing-bed program, even for SNF patients alone (i.e., excluding ICF patients), on the premise that they would be paying more providers for nursing home care. However, the success of the swing-bed program suggests that state Medicaid programs may be able to further save money, especially for patients who are not yet eligible for Medicare (i.e., not yet 65) but need near-acute care after discharge from an acute care hospital.

Out of justifiable concerns that budgets are never adequate, state Medicaid programs and legislatures are continually seeking ways to have their costs underwritten by health care providers and other payers, including private payers. This is done in a variety of ways in the acute care, long-term care, and ambulatory care fields. It was noted earlier that increased Medicare SNF coverage under the Medicare Catastrophic Coverage Act of 1988 resulted in some state Medicaid programs building an expected savings into their budget as a result of Medicare's underwriting more SNF care for chronic care patients that Medicaid previously had covered. The budgetary problems for these states were exacerbated when the act was repealed. While this type of thinking is not unreasonable, it can cause serious problems. In the case of the swing-bed program, it inhibited state Medicaid programs from venturing into an innovative type of care that is probably as cost-effective for Medicaid as it is for Medicare.

In our long-term care system at large, federal dollars under Medicaid are channeled through individual states. The federal government does not have the power to require states to adopt specific courses and directions. Congress determined that states should have responsibility for shaping their own programs. Currently, we see a relatively fragmented approach to the provision of long-term care for the poor or near poor under state Medicaid programs that are preoccupied with balancing budgets by implicitly and even explicitly taking the behavior of various public and private payers into consideration in determining their payment policies. We are still learning about the phenomena of Medicaid eligibility for, and utilization patterns associated with, nursing home care (Liu, Doty, and Manton 1990; Moses 1990; Spence and Wiener 1990). The origins of Medicare in acute care and Medicaid in more traditional or chronic long-term care, and the different nature of their beneficiaries, have resulted in the programs too frequently working at odds rather than complementarily. These issues not only deserve attention nationally, but they must be continually borne in mind when structuring any type of change in long-term care reimbursement policies.

Is a Comprehensive Long-Term Care Policy Essential to Improve Near-Acute Care?

While the Medicare-Medicaid interrelation dilemma is a serious one, it only partially highlights the complex nature of the problems of our long-term care delivery system. Nationally, nursing home costs (21 percent of hospital costs in 1986) have grown approximately 50 percent more rapidly than hospital costs since 1965 (NCHS 1988). The costs of non-institutional long-term care, and especially care provided by family and friends, are truly massive. Depending on how one defines long-term care and whether one is concerned about direct costs to payers versus the more indirect costs to society incurred by family and friends providing various types of support and health care services, it can be argued that long-term care is the most costly component of our extended health care delivery system in the United States.

In a public policy context, we must determine the following:

— how much institutional versus noninstitutional long-term care we should be providing

— how much and what types of long-term care currently being provided by family and friends should or should not be supported with public funds

— how to better integrate acute care and long-term care from the perspective of cost and quality

— how to structure our major public financing programs for long-term care so they do not work at cross purposes or provide disincentives to innovate

— how to encourage private financing in the long-term care field

— perhaps more importantly, which services are essential for what types of patients according to some policy-determined priority scheme based on need and cost effectiveness of services

Others have begun to articulate a broad policy of long-term care (or health care in general) in the United States, including financing approaches (Rivlin et al. 1988; IOM 1986; Moon 1989; Kane 1990; Hughes 1986; Eisendorfer, Kessler, and Spector 1989; Ball 1990; Gist 1989; Shortell and McNerney 1990; Smeeding 1990). The Pepper Commission, established under the Medicare Catastrophic Coverage Act, also put forth a rather sweeping set of recommendations for our long-term care delivery system. Such proposals and platforms are clearly necessary since they force us to consider policy trade-offs in a variety of different ways. On the other hand, as Merrill and Somers (1989) said in their aptly named article, "Long-Term Care: The Great Debate on the Wrong Issue," we need an infrastructure to serve as a foundation on which to superimpose or build a changed approach to delivering, financing, and regulating long-term care in the United States. Thus, as important as recommendations for financing or refinancing our long-term care system might be, and we already have a number of well–thought out options in this regard, we need reasonably specific recommendations on how our long-term care system should be structured and integrated before a comprehensive long-term care policy can be thoroughly articulated.

In deliberations on financing and reimbursement in the long-term care field, capitated approaches are raised with far greater frequency than in the past. We have to be careful not to see capitation as a comprehensive short-run answer to all problems in the health care field. For example, we have a growing tendency to simply adopt the posture that if we bundle large groups of services together and reimburse through some form of capitation (i.e., pay for a patient with a single lump sum that would cover a preset time interval of care regardless of who provides it—or even cover a single year), that everything will be fine. If the services for which we are capitating are well-defined and highly integrated, with no quality-of-care problems, this is a reasonable approach. However, at times we fail to recognize that we are making these assumptions, especially with respect to quality of care or patient outcomes, in advocating capitation on a more widespread basis. While most of us are proponents of capitated payment under many circumstances, we cannot allow such circumstances to include instances where we are not certain how we should provide care, where we are unclear on who should provide it, and when there is a reasonable chance that we have problems with respect to quality of care. We cannot "black box" problems by simply "letting the industry take care of it." Rather we must exert a concentrated effort to be certain that integration, and adequate services and outcomes, are assured. In many areas of health care, we have little choice but to proceed on a more incremental basis rather than simply make wholesale changes from a reimbursement or financing perspective on the assumption that all the patient care pieces will simply fall into place. At this stage of evolution of our health care system, it would be irresponsible to implement large-scale, wholesale changes in reimbursement policy that assume our existing system is adequate in assessing the need for and providing long-term care.

It would be wonderful if we could implement a set of sweeping changes in long-term care that would result in a comprehensive, integrated, high-quality, and well-financed system of long-term care in the United States. In all likelihood, we will continue to struggle for many years to, at best, approximate this objective. To be able to make inroads in specific areas of long-term care, such as near-acute care, should be regarded as well worth an investment of resources. There is no way we can possibly overhaul our long-term care system with one sweeping set of changes. Our system is far too complex, and as demand for care, types of care needs, and care technologies change over time, we have to continually adapt and reevaluate.

CHAPTER 7 SUMMARY

Several policy initiatives implemented in the 1970s and early 1980s resulted in pronounced changes in the types and care needs of patients in nursing homes, home health agencies, and hospitals. Nursing homes that care for high proportions of Medicare patients experienced a substantial increase in the medical, skilled nursing, and therapeutic needs of their patients. More traditional nursing homes that care predominantly for Medicaid and private-pay patients witnessed a strong increase in the functional care needs (e.g., bathing, dressing, feeding) of patients. Medicare-certified home health agencies experienced a pronounced increase in functional needs of their patients and, to a lesser extent, certain types of skilled nursing and therapy needs. Because some types of patients who had previously been hospitalized were no longer treated on an inpatient basis, our hospital care system experienced a general increase in the acute care needs of its patients.

The policy-related causes of what was probably the most dramatic case-mix increase in the history of our health care system were severalfold. Without doubt, PPS altered the nature of hospital care, providing incentives for shorter stays and more intense acuity levels on a per day or average-stay basis for hospital patients. Since such patients were discharged sooner, nursing homes and home health agencies generally experienced an increase in near-acute care needs of posthospital patients. In the late 1970s and early 1980s, the deinstitutionalization movement for nursing homes resulted in more stringent Medicaid preadmission screening programs throughout the country. These were targeted at avoiding institutionalization for patients who were judged sufficiently independent to function at home or in other less intense care settings. These programs frequently accompanied home- and community-based care alternatives in many states. When combined with the impacts of PPS that resulted in more posthospital patients with near-acute care needs, these state-initiated policy changes substantially increased the case-mix intensity of home health care patients. Due to a liberalization of the Medicare benefit for home health care in 1980, the number of

Medicare-certified home health agencies increased greatly during the first half of the 1980s.

Overall, our combined acute care and long-term care system experienced a powerful set of changes to which we are still acclimating. In conjunction with an equally strong set of changes about to occur in physician reimbursement under Medicare, it is apparent that it will take us well into the 1990s, very likely until the turn of the century, to improve our approaches to coordinating and integrating acute care, long-term care, and ambulatory/outpatient care. Not only will reimbursement and access issues require continued scrutiny and appropriate modification, but quality of health care will continue to be of paramount importance. We must continue to address whether the changes we have brought about (with noble intentions from the perspective of both cost control and access) are overtaxing certain segments of our health care system—to the point where quality of care is suffering. In certain areas, it is likely that quality of care was not adequate to start with and that we have exacerbated our problems with our changes. In others, we may have remedied some of our problems by the significant changes made in Medicare reimbursement. In yet other ways, we may have inadvertently created new problems through our reimbursement system changes. We need to objectively assess the best ways to integrate acute care, long-term care, and ambulatory/outpatient care purely from the perspective of patient care—independently of how we pay for such care. In addition, we should specify the appropriate models for integration and coordination, and determine how closely we can approximate them in view of what we can afford.

Near-acute care is an important fulcrum in coordinating acute, long-term, and ambulatory/outpatient care. Patients in need of near-acute care are often, but not always, posthospital long-term care patients with relatively short-term needs. They may require posthospital institutional care, noninstitutional home-based or ambulatory/outpatient care, or both to attain their rehabilitation potential. During the 1980s, the terms *subacute care* and *transitional care* were used to refer to care often provided to patients with near-acute care problems. Subacute care usually connotes relatively intense long-term care provided to patients with above-average medical and skilled nursing needs. Yet, it is defined differently by various state Medicaid programs, and in some circles, the term *subacute care* refers to any type of care that is "below" acute care— referring to almost all types of long-term care. The term *transitional care* typically refers to care provided in assisting with the transition from acute care to other types of health care. At times, PPS-exempt rehabilitation hospitals, especially when they exist as a distinct unit within a short-term general hospital, are referred to as *transitional care units*. Because of different meanings associated with these terms, *near-acute care* has been introduced in this book to connote "short-term" care typically provided to long-term care patients with relatively pronounced skilled nursing, medical, and therapeutic care needs.

Since the early 1980s, we have been attempting to come to grips with how best to provide, pay for, and regulate near-acute care, particularly in metropolitan areas. Hospitals do not wish to provide such care in hospital beds with no or inadequate reimbursement. Yet, nursing homes and other long-term care providers often do not have the capacity to provide care to such patients. Near-acute care patients are sometimes discharged to inappropriate settings or retained in hospital beds where either reimbursement or care may be inadequate for patient needs. When discharged to a traditional nursing home—if a nursing home will admit such patients—coordination between the acute care providers and the long-term care providers, as well as continual assessment and monitoring of patient needs with a view toward rehabilitation and discharge to independent living, can be inadequate. In many rural communities, however, where approximately 1,200 hospitals implemented the swing-bed approach in the 1980s, this problem is less pronounced. Near-acute care patients are retained in the hospital in swing beds, with the hospital receiving Medicare reimbursement for long-term care and patients benefiting from the acute care environment of the hospital, which typically has the needed staff and equipment present to provide near-acute care. Patients are not transferred to acute care even in various instances where nursing home patients would otherwise be transferred to a hospital, with the transfer often increasing both trauma to the patient and cost to payers. Nevertheless, since the majority of health care in this country is provided in metropolitan areas, we are confronted with the issue of how best to provide such care nationally. The swing-bed approach appears to be a significant portion of the solution in rural areas, but has not yet been tried in metropolitan areas. The issues of access to, payment for, and quality of near-acute care are serious ones in the United States.

Several other events and practices during the 1980s shed light on how we might proceed with structuring, coordinating, and providing near-acute care. For example, in the 1960s and 1970s it had been conjectured that there was little room for substitution of long-term care for acute care. Programs that were researched in the 1980s, however, have given us a clear basis for refuting this hypothesis. Not only was it apparent that long-term care provided in hospital swing beds had the capacity to reduce the use of acute care, but feasibility studies and demonstration projects in the areas of teaching nursing homes and the use of geriatric nurse practitioners showed that well-provided long-term care can reduce the use of hospital care. An experiment in which nursing home patients who experienced a sudden decline in health status were cared for in well-equipped nursing homes with far more physician care than is frequently available for nursing home patients demonstrated a significant cost savings by substituting such care for acute care services.

The field of geriatric assessment and treatment grew during the 1980s (although it is still far from widespread in the United States). Some of our geriatric assessment and treatment programs bear promise for enhanced patient outcomes and reduced use of acute care services. Geriatric assessment typically refers to a comprehensive assessment of a patient's needs conducted by an interdisciplinary team of providers. While the jury is out on the specific types of patients for which geriatric assessment might be cost-effective, there is at least some cause for optimism about the potential benefits of targeting selected patient types for geriatric assessment services. Other programs have been implemented by various providers to better coordinate and integrate acute care and long-term care services, often focusing on near-acute care as a reasonable starting point for such integration. Some of these programs are funded by external agencies, while others have been initiated by individual providers. To date, however, no major changes in reimbursement policy have been undertaken to test and assess cost effectiveness of financial incentives in changing provider behavior in the area of near-acute care.

In general, the provider settings and programs that have been reasonably successful in providing near-acute care, by reducing acute care and enhancing patient outcomes, appear to have several common features. First, some form of reasonably comprehensive assessment involving a provider team consisting of at least a physician and skilled nurse, often augmented by a therapist, social worker, or both, depending on patient needs, has marked the initiation of the care program for near-acute care patients. Second, most successful approaches have involved relatively close monitoring of patient status and the care plan, which is updated with appropriate changes. Third, a systematic means of coordinating and integrating the various types of care the near-acute care patient requires has been manifest, at times in the form of a single individual who might be termed the *care coordinator*. This individual is typically knowledgeable about and experienced in medical care or skilled nursing care, and often a member of the medical/skilled nursing care team that cares for the near-acute care patient. Fourth, considerably greater involvement on the part of physicians is apparent (than for more traditional long-term care patients). Fifth, the most successful experiences appear to have involved patient selection, targeting near-acute care patients with rehabilitation potential.

The enactment and repeal of the Medicare Catastrophic Coverage Act of 1988 brought about a brief period of involvement by Medicare in the more traditional long-term care field, largely by extending the Medicare SNF benefit to cover longer nursing home stays. Medicare expenditures on SNF care increased threefold during the roughly one-year period while the new benefit was in place, although this may have been due as much to revised coverage guidelines for Medicare SNF care that were implemented almost coterminously with the Catastrophic Coverage Act. Whether and how soon the Medicare SNF benefit might again be changed to cover longer stays remains to be seen. However, many think Medicare does not belong in the traditional long-term care field, rather this is the domain of Medicaid. In any event, the type of alteration required in the Medicare SNF benefit for near-acute care patients would certainly not bring Medicare closer to the domain of traditional long-term care. Rather, near-acute care tends to focus exclusively on more intense types of Medicare SNF care and possibly certain types of PPS-exempt rehabilitation care.

The rural swing-bed program was extended to larger hospitals (less than 100 beds) in 1987, although it is presently unclear whether this more restrictive approach to providing hospital swing-bed care in larger hospitals will assist us in addressing our near-acute care dilemma nationally. Since the secretary of the Department of Health and Human Services has demonstration authority under the Omnibus Budget Reconciliation Act of 1980 to experiment with the swing-bed approach in metropolitan areas, it appears plausible to assess the potential cost effectiveness of providing swing-bed care in larger urban hospitals on an experimental basis.

In considering options for restructuring near-acute care, several policy considerations are relevant. First, near-acute care can be successfully provided in a number of different settings, including "super" SNFs (i.e., Medicare-certified nursing homes that are well-equipped to provide near-acute care); more traditional Medicare SNFs—both hospital-based and, at times, freestanding SNFs; some certified home health agencies that provide relatively high-tech services; swing-bed hospitals; PPS-exempt rehabilitation hospitals that typically provide care to near-acute patients that can endure extremely intensive therapy over a short period of time; and through administratively necessary days provisions that allow hospitals to provide near-acute care in acute care beds under some state Medicaid programs. In all, our approach to providing near-acute care nationally, however, has been fragmented, has evolved in a piecemeal fashion, and is presently not well integrated either in terms of patient care or providers involved in such care.

Second, while we now have a reasonable base of knowledge of the essential ingredients for cost-effective near-acute care for patients with rehabilitation potential on which to build, we must examine closely which provider settings are most appropriate and how to coordinate such care across provider settings. In the process of doing this, as was the case with swing-bed care in rural communities, we must recognize that we cannot be overly rigid in regulating such care, at least under circumstances where we are trying to innovate. Flexible regulation is important.

Third, we have understandable fears that larger hospitals with their more sophisticated administrative and financial staff, as well as their higher cost structures, might unnecessarily increase the cost of near-acute care if it were provided in a hospital setting. However, we must recognize and objectively assess the potential represented by empty hospital beds in the United States, particularly if we properly incorporate financial disincentives or regulatory safeguards to prevent such potential abuses. Near-acute care provided in such beds may prove to be cost-effective even in larger urban hospitals. The rural experience with hospital swing beds, however, does not guarantee success in urban areas.

Fourth, it may be possible to bundle reimbursement for near-acute care in various ways. If a near-acute care stay is provided in an institutional setting, it may be appropriate ultimately to pay the institution a lump sum for the provision of all near-acute care provided to the patient, regardless of whether different providers may be involved in such care. Thus, it is possible that an approach analogous to DRGs for Medicare acute care (i.e., under PPS) may be possible for near-acute care. In fact, it is quite likely. Although close, we are not yet at the point where enough information is available to structure an equitable and effective reimbursement approach in this regard. It is important to recall that near-acute care is a type of long-term care and, as such, is radically different from acute care in terms of the ability to forecast patient resource needs as a function of diagnoses. Other patient conditions better forecast resource needs. To date, some consideration has been given to bundling acute care and long-term care services strictly on the basis of DRGs, adding a certain amount to hospital reimbursement to cover postacute care for at least selected types of patients. Although the idea has merit from the perspective of consolidated reimbursement and integrating long-term care and acute care, we are far from being able to forecast long-term care needs on the basis of acute care diagnoses and procedures. Nevertheless, service and payment bundling may be viable over the long term. If properly structured, they can provide incentives for improved service coordination and integration. We must be fully cognizant, however, of precisely what services are appropriate and necessary for near-acute care patients before we implement a bundling approach nationally, since quality of, or access to, care can be seriously impaired if we do not have a clear sense of the infrastructure of this emerging subfield within long-term care.

Fifth, from a policy perspective, it is evident that incentives for increased involvement on the part of physicians are important for improved near-acute care in the United States. In all likelihood, this means we should be willing to pay for increased physician visits to such patients since it will both enhance patient well-being and reduce the overall costs of care, particularly acute care resulting from unnecessary readmissions to hospitals.

Lastly, over the past several years we have witnessed a number of well–thought out proposals on how best to finance long-term care in the United States. Many of these proposals and approaches are insightful and bear considerable merit. We will doubtlessly implement one or more of these proposals in some modified form as we work through the intricacies of financing long-term care over the course of the 1990s, building on our experiences and recommendations of the 1980s. Equally important, however, and possibly even more important, are (1) the issues associated with how best to structure and integrate our various types of long-term care, and (2) how best to structure and integrate the entire spectrum of care ranging from acute care to long-term care to outpatient/ambulatory care (including many other types of services such as mental health services, etc.) under our health care system as it exists in the United States. We have an astonishingly wide variety of payment mechanisms and consumer choices. It is unlikely that this variation will be substantially diminished even over the next 20 to 30 years because of the nature of our society and our economic system. We must recognize that the total dollars that we spend, and even the way we allocate these dollars, must be invested in a logical and well-integrated infrastructure for the provision of health care services. We need a focal point to begin the task of systematically analyzing and integrating such an infrastructure. Near-acute care can be this focal point.

CHAPTER 8

What We Have Learned and What We Should Do in Shaping Policy for Near-Acute Care

Since this chapter is intended to be more comprehensively read than preceding chapters, an effort has been made to avoid technical material. Salient points raised in preceding chapters are reiterated here. My intent is to synthesize, draw conclusions, and propose future directions to pursue in addressing selected policy issues, particularly those relating to near-acute care. The technical information that supports the points made in this chapter can be found in earlier chapters, where the chapter summaries provide an overview of the basic conclusions reached.

POLICY FORMULATION LESSONS LEARNED FROM THE SWING-BED EXPERIENCE

Health Care Providers Do Best What Comes Naturally

Time and again in evaluating the swing-bed program, we saw and heard people expressing concerns that long-term care could not be adequately provided in hospital swing beds. Representatives of the nursing home industry argued that hospital staff are not trained or oriented to provide institutional long-term care. Hospital nursing staff expressed the concern that they did not want their hospitals to become nursing homes. Hospital administrators complained it would not work because of low volume and inadequate reimbursement. Physicians were frequently lukewarm about the provision of nursing home care in hospital beds. State regulatory personnel representing certification programs and certificate-of-need programs were reluctant to endorse the swing-bed approach because it opened the equivalent of more nursing home beds, possibly in facilities that would not be able to do as good a job as nursing homes. Medicare and Medicaid program officials expressed the concern that swing-bed care would cost more than nursing home care, and later that providers would game the reimbursement system under the prospective payment system (PPS). They were concerned that hospitals would double-dip by collecting first a per case payment upon early discharge from acute care, then a per day payment for each day of swing-bed care, followed by another per case payment for a second Medicare-covered acute care stay for another diagnosis-related group (DRG). Further, they could minimize ancillary services during the acute care stay and receive cost-based reimbursement for such services during the swing-bed stay.

Virtually none of these concerns were realized. Why? The warnings were logical and well-founded in terms of financial incentives and provider-related concerns. What appears to have happened is that the staff of swing-bed hospitals became aware of the significant need for near-acute care in their respective rural communities and simply provided such care exceptionally well—better than rural nursing homes. On the other hand, they tended not to get into the business of providing traditional nursing home care to long-stay patients (although this was done in a few swing-bed hospitals). They typically gravitated toward providing a type of care that was more medically intense and required skilled services that were available in hospital settings, doing so extremely well. The results demonstrate that providers respond to more than purely financial incentives. Reimbursement was considered marginally adequate, or at least not terribly inadequate, in the eyes of hospital administrative staff, to the point where it was seen as nearly sufficient for covering the cost of a program that was clearly beneficial to the community. Reimbursement system abuses occurred in highly isolated cases, but double-dipping did not generally occur. Furthermore, it turned out that Medicare was saving money. Costs to Medicare (and probably Medicaid) were reduced in two ways. First, the average per day rates paid under the swing-bed program were lower than nursing home rates, especially for Medicare patients. Yet, the swing-bed approach helped avoid building new nursing homes in various locations. Second, reduced rehospitalization rates and reduced use of outpatient care by Medicare patients resulted in lower per capita health care costs for Medicare beneficiaries admitted to swing-bed hospitals.

This "naturalness approach" of giving providers sufficient flexibility to provide the care that they are capable of providing (somewhat in their own way) appears to have been one of the primary reasons for the success of the swing-bed program. In retrospect, it became apparent that acute care providers were not about to veer substantially from their chosen direction or natural instincts as providers of health care for a relatively small program (that would nonetheless be of substantial benefit to their community). Although strong, the need for near-acute care in rural communities was well circumscribed. Generally speaking, hospital staff and administration did not want to go beyond this need and compete directly with nursing homes for traditional long-term care patients. Instead they admitted patients in need of long-term care services, assessing such needs and providing rehabilitation/restorative services to the extent they were available through the hospital environment. Most patients did not stay beyond three weeks. The proportion of patients rehabilitated was considerably greater than would typically be the case for similar patients admitted to rural nursing homes. Some patients required chronic care in traditional nursing homes and were therefore discharged to such facilities. In all, a type of care was provided that was natural for hospital staff to provide to long-term care patients in hospital beds, namely near-acute care. The national swing-bed program proved remarkably successful in providing such care from the perspectives of quality, cost, and overall effectiveness. The lesson learned: innovations in the health care field, where possible, should be built on extant provider strengths, allowing some degree of flexibility for new programs to naturally evolve on the basis of such strengths.

A Scientific Approach to Policy Is Possible

In the autumn of 1969, the swing-bed program began as an idea in Bruce Walter's mind. He advocated experimenting with this approach to providing long-term care in acute care hospital beds in the early 1970s, successfully convincing the Department of Health, Education, and Welfare to fund a demonstration project in rural Utah. In view of the findings from the evaluations of the Utah demonstration and the ensuing demonstrations in Texas, Iowa, and South Dakota, the overall cost effectiveness of the swing-bed approach in rural communities became apparent. As a result of the experience with the demonstrations and the results from the evaluation studies, both Congress and the administration took note of and supported the swing-bed approach by the late 1970s. A number of bills were introduced supporting swing-bed care nationally, and associated testimony was heard during 1978 and 1979. Finally, the Omnibus Budget Reconciliation Act of 1980 contained the enabling legislation for a national swing-bed program in rural hospitals.

On the basis of the experience with the demonstration and evaluation programs in the 1970s, the Robert Wood Johnson Foundation (RWJF) funded a model program designed to assist rural hospitals throughout the country in implementing swing beds. Twenty-six hospitals in five states received grants to undertake swing-bed care on a more accelerated basis. They were supported by their state hospital associations, who also received grants and promulgated information on their experiences. The Health Care Financing Administration's evaluation study of the national program and the RWJF study of their model program in the mid-1980s showed that the national program took hold slowly, but its ultimate expansion and success was due largely to four factors.

First, for the same reason that the demonstration program was successful in the 1970s (i.e., the naturalness approach mentioned above), the program eventually settled in nationally. Simply put, it capitalized on the strength of small hospitals to provide near-acute long-term care. Second, the information promulgated to interested hospitals and communities on the basis of the prior demonstrations and the RWJF model program served as a practical springboard for hospital staff interested in implementing a swing-bed program in their community hospitals. Third, PPS was a catalyst for hospitals to initiate the swing-bed approach in the mid-1980s. Such hospitals were able to take advantage of the information base and experience already available from the pioneering hospitals in the early 1980s. Fourth, a genuine community need existed for the near-acute care services that rural swing-bed hospitals could provide to long-term care patients. Combined with regulatory flexibility and a straightforward, but not overly generous, approach to reimbursement for swing-bed care, the program took hold in such a manner as to meet this community need, but provided few real incentives for overutilization or reimbursement maximization.

Thus, the swing-bed approach that involves over 1,200 hospitals at this writing began as a modest experimental program with 25 hospitals in rural Utah. By virtue of study, refinement, and an evolution characterized by disseminating information on what worked and what did not work with this approach in rural communities, we now have a highly beneficial program meeting a community need for near-acute care in a large number of rural communities throughout the United States. The track record of the program demonstrates that it is possible to refine and constructively influence health policy through an objective approach to experimentation and research on how to provide health services.

Evolution-Shaping Demonstration Programs Can Work

The prominence that the swing-bed approach received through the RWJF model program was considerable. The key problems that hospitals, payers, regulators, and communities were likely to encounter were discussed, and solutions promulgated, prior to and during implementation of the swing-bed approach throughout the country. In late 1983, a time when controversy surrounding reimbursement for acute care painted an exceptionally bleak picture for rural hospitals, 101 of the 149 swing-bed hospitals participating in the national program were either RWJF grantee hospitals or prior HCFA demonstration hospitals from the late 1970s. The visibility resulting from the RWJF program contributed to sustaining the swing-bed approach during this period. Within three years, the size of the national program had increased to nearly 900 hospitals.

Due in part to the implementation of PPS, the almost exponential growth of the program nationally between 1983 and 1987 had the potential to disrupt the provision of acute care and long-term care in rural communities, weaken the quality of long-term care in such communities, cause serious problems for payers and regulators, and result in considerable gaming of Medicare reimbursement by rural hospitals. Yet few of these problems occurred. While PPS represented an incentive for hospitals to be interested in swing-bed care, significant communication, planning, and implementation vehicles for the swing-bed approach were provided by the RWJF program and the American Hospital Association–sponsored activities that accompanied it. In fact, it appears that a number of pitfalls regarding quality assurance, reimbursement, and integration with extant long-term care providers were avoided as the program grew and took hold. The model program funded by RWJF played a major role as a precursor to the large-scale national program now in place throughout the country. By almost any standards, the growth of the swing-bed program in rural communities throughout the country was unusually trouble-free and well administered at the community, state, regional, and federal levels.

New approaches to delivering health care at the national level are often brought about by regulatory and reimbursement changes, frequently through legislation. Significant policy changes in reimbursement and regulation therefore signify either the start of a new approach to providing health care or a substantial deviation in current approaches. For example, the regulatory and reimbursement policy changes embodied in Section 904 of OBRA 1980 provided the basis for, and signified the implementation of, the national swing-bed program. Analogously, the major thrust of PPS was embodied in legislation that signified a substantial change in hospital reimbursement and, as a corollary, a major change in the practice of providing hospital inpatient care. As a third example, a significant change in the Medicare home health benefit in the early 1980s not only brought about a large increase in the number of home health providers, but it also radically changed the manner in which home health care is now provided at a national level.

Prior to implementing such changes or new programs, demonstrations or research programs have often been conducted, pointing to or negating the feasibility of the approach on a more widespread basis. However, despite the value of such demonstrations in determining the likelihood of program effectiveness, the circumstances surrounding demonstrations necessarily precede, and are therefore different from, those that will accompany implementation of a new national program or a sweeping change in an extant program. The effectiveness of the RWJF model program at the outset of implementing the national swing-bed program points to the utility of another type of demonstration that can assist in guiding the evolution of a national program concurrent with its implementation. An evolution-shaping demonstration of this nature appears to have practical utility. Two important attributes of this type of an evolution-shaping demonstration are the speed with which it is implemented at the outset of a major program change and the extent of information dissemination to assist other providers, regulators, and payers in resolving problems and forming policies.

This approach to demonstration programs should be considered on a more widespread basis. For example, even though HCFA did fund demonstrations in some states prior to PPS, if a number of hospitals throughout the country had been funded at the *outset* of PPS to implement model record keeping, utilization review, and quality assurance programs in view of the radical changes that PPS would bring about, such a demonstration may have greatly facilitated and even altered the path that hospital care and quality assurance have taken under PPS. The potential for evolution-shaping demonstrations to guide and constructively alter the direction taken by major health care programs appears to be substantial.

Incrementalism Works

In keeping with the axiom "the longer the time, the finer the wine," it took a considerable period of time, between ten and twenty years, for the swing-bed approach to evolve into a program that now meets the near-acute care needs of a large number of rural communities. It is easy to say that if in the early 1970s we had simply implemented a program with all the characteristics of our current national approach to providing swing-bed care, we could have accomplished sooner what took almost two decades to accomplish. But we had no crystal ball, nor did we have any clear idea of how the program would evolve nationally. Its earliest proponents saw it as a means of providing traditional long-term care in hospital beds. This was exemplified by the lengths of stay for patients receiving swing-bed care under the original Utah demonstration, which were comparable to those of nursing home patients in Utah at that time.

The original average stays of between 250 and 300 days were more than ten times greater than the average stays of two to three weeks that now characterize the national swing-bed program. In fact, the original Utah program was conceived and implemented primarily as a program to meet more traditional chronic long-term care needs of residents of rural communities. In this regard, the Utah experience was atypical.

The ensuing demonstrations in Iowa, South Dakota, and Texas saw the patient care emphasis shift to shorter-stay patients who did not have the traditional chronic care needs of nursing home patients. A modified reimbursement approach was used in the central Iowa demonstration, which eventually formed the basis for reimbursement under the national program. The experience in dealing with extant regulatory requirements and programs, including certificate-of-need and certification policies, contributed to shaping how the swing-bed approach should be integrated with various public-payer requirements that must accompany any national program. In fact, it is now clear that if we had simply slammed the swing-bed program into place nationally in the early 1970s as it was originally designed, it probably would have been quite useless. It would have simply represented another approach to providing traditional long-term care, but in a provider setting that was not as conducive to providing such care as nursing homes. The quality of care and quality of life for long-stay patients would have been inadequate, and community needs for near-acute care probably would not have been satisfied with the same efficacy that now characterizes the swing-bed program nationally. Further, the program might have been totally stymied from a regulatory perspective; the Medicare and Medicaid conditions of participation that were waived would have been ultimately enforced since they represent basic structural quality standards relevant to more traditional long-term care patients. The vast majority of rural hospitals would not have invested the resources necessary to comply with such standards.

Yes, the evolution of the program was slow. Some of us would have liked it to proceed more quickly, especially after we became reasonably familiar with how it would and would not work. But many patients ultimately benefited considerably from the time it took to evolve. Those of us in the health policy field often feel that an incremental approach to building and shaping health policy is, at a minimum, inefficient. However, it seems to have produced admirably positive results in this case. A "big bang" approach to implementing swing beds nationally without experimentation and research would likely have fallen on its face.

This is not to say that incrementalism is always appropriate. It is not necessary to research every single type of health care program that warrants national attention. Rather, in circumstances where we do not have an adequate idea of the course an innovation might follow, and when the approach appears to have merit, it makes sense to slow down for a few years to assess how we might benefit optimally from the program in terms of both cost and effectiveness. Historically, HCFA has conducted a number of useful demonstrations of this type, and over the last ten years Congress has also been mandating more research undertakings of this nature.

Impediments to Overcome in Rationally Setting Policy

Our research on hospital swing beds and other selected programs that led to policy change or formulation points out several naturally occurring impediments to policy change. First, providers are typically hesitant to innovate, especially when a new type of care is required of the provider and when reimbursement for that type of care is different from what the provider typically experiences. The two biggest impediments to overcome in the swing-bed program at the hospital level were (1) the hesitancy of hospital staff to become involved in providing long-term care in acute care beds, and (2) the general resistance to reimbursement that, by the industry's definition, would probably be inadequate since it would come from Medicare and Medicaid (and since it was based on reimbursement for nursing homes in the first place). Further, many providers, including hospitals and some types of physicians, are presently confronted with a highly antagonistic reimbursement climate (in their opinion). Anything Medicare and Medicaid try to do is suspect. The heyday of hospital growth, the 1940s, 1950s, and 1960s, and of widespread cost-based reimbursement by public (and commercial) payers, the 1970s, is over. In some ways the world of public and commercial payers is now flailing about trying to control the cost-eating monsters of hospital care and ambulatory care that it created. In this environment, hospital staff and physicians will not immediately espouse public sector regulatory or reimbursement innovations; they first must prove to be useful from a provider perspective. Until proven innocent, such innovations will be judged guilty of inappropriate intrusion and financial deprivation.

Innovation aimed at increasing the flexibility of regulatory and reimbursement policy often strikes at the very heart of the bureaucracy we have established to administer our publicly sponsored health care programs in the United States (and to regulate health care in general). After 25 years of Medicare and Medicaid, we have now developed a complex network of organizations and suborganizations that administer these programs, accompanied by an equally complex network of rules, regulations, practices, and even unspoken customs and traditions that are integrally and confusingly entangled. The extent of similarities and differences in state Medicaid programs is mind-boggling. The differences with which federal rules and regulations are implemented, interpreted, and enforced by regional offices, fiscal intermediaries, certification agencies, surveyors, review agency staff, new versus extant PROs, etc., is at times depressing. Yet the system goes on. It is essential we acknowledge, however, that we need these various functions and that it is not easy to administer massive programs of the nature of Medicare and Medicaid.

The intent here is not to suggest how to improve these programs organizationally (since this is not my area of expertise). Rather, we must expect that in a bureaucracy as comprehensive and as complex as that which now administers our publicly financed health care programs in the United States, we will understandably encounter serious resistance to innovation of various types. For example, in some states it is now clear that the staff of PROs and certification agencies are truly unaware of the value of the swing-bed approach nationally. I have given presentations at various workshops and meetings throughout the country on swing-bed care and continue to discuss swing-bed issues with provider representatives, regulators, and payers on a frequent basis. The bureaucratic rules and regulations that characterize review agencies, certification agencies, and so on, simply dictate that it is their job at times to attempt to find problems and stymie certain types of activities. At times it is difficult for them to take the stance that innovation *might* bring about greater efficiency or *might* increase the quality of care. It is important to add, however, that staff have been encountered in a number of such agencies who routinely take the high road and support innovation. Nonetheless, resistance of the nature discussed is not unusual. Those committed to innovation should regard such resistance as natural and, just as in the case of provider resistance, regard it as a phenomenon with which one must constructively deal.

According to a knowledgeable and competent colleague at HCFA, "the swing-bed program is little more than a rounding error in the Medicare budget." On the one hand, this statement is not too far from true when you look at the total 1985 Medicare budget of $69.3 billion (Letsch, Levit, and Waldo 1988) compared with total Medicare expenditures on swing-bed care of $26.1 million in 1985 (Shaughnessy, Schlenker, et al. 1989b). On the other hand, when we break the various types of health care we provide into reasonably small parcels, this can be said about almost any type of health care. Surely the tens of thousands of residents of rural communities who have benefited from the swing-bed program do not think it is inconsequential. Further, in view of the potential improvements in our health care system that are now suggested on the basis of the swing-bed approach, it is far from inconsequential from a policy perspective. Although this potential is discussed later, the main concern here is with the apparent smallness of most (but not all) innovations when compared with the totality of our health care system. If any approach to improving health care is cost effective (i.e., its benefits outweigh its costs relative to the status quo), it warrants attention. The decade of the 1980s, especially with the understandable emphasis placed on PPS, might be termed the decade where the acute care tail wagged the entire health care delivery system dog. Important interrelationships among various aspects of our health care system cannot and should not be overlooked. Innovation and change in one area, for example, acute care, ultimately precipitates change in others areas.

CONSIDERATIONS INVOLVED IN IMPROVING NEAR-ACUTE LONG-TERM CARE

Near-Acute Care

As discussed in Chapter 7, the phrases "transitional care," "alternate level of care," and "subacute care" were introduced in the 1980s to connote hard-to-find long-term care needed by patients discharged from hospitals. With shorter hospital stays and increased near-acute care needs of patients discharged from hospitals under PPS, our hospital care system encountered a substantial increase in patients who could not be easily placed in long-term care settings. *Transitional care* and *alternate level of care* are now used in a variety of ways. Often these terms are used to connote care for any types of hospital patients that are hard to place in long-term care settings. Other times they refer to long-term care for postacute patients with intense medical needs. *Subacute care* at times is intended to mean long-term care that is not necessarily postacute but is reasonably intense in terms of medical and skilled nursing care. However, subacute care can be used to refer to any type of long-term care that is less complex than acute care. In this book, the term has this broad meaning—that is, any type of long-term care that is less resource-intensive than acute care.

For the sake of clarity and to avoid confusion with other terms that have multiple meanings (including different meanings in different states), the term *near-acute care patients* has been introduced to refer to patients whose long-term care needs are relatively intense from a medical and skilled nursing perspective. No attempt is made to define near-acute care rigorously here—this is best left up to regulators in conjunction with patient care experts. In general, however, near-acute care refers to a level of long-term care that is not acute care, but normally requires more intensive skilled nursing and medical care than is typically provided in a skilled nursing facility. A near-acute patient does not have to be a posthospital patient, nor does the patient have to have strong rehabilitation potential. The successes that have been encountered with the provision of near-acute care, however, have typically involved patients that have rehabilitation potential.

The Goal: An Integrated System of Care

We often talk of a "continuum of care" that ranges from acute care through a variety of different types of subacute care (in the broad sense). As discussed in Chapter 7, there very likely is no such long-term care continuum (Vladeck 1987b), particularly from the perspective of cost or resource consumption, although there may be from the perspective of professional provider skills and technology required. Regardless, too infrequently do we talk about how best to integrate the main types of subacute care or the main patient transition points among the range of subacute care providers (Evashwick and Weiss 1987; Bowlyow 1990). Acute care patients are often discharged to other care environments with inadequate assessment, inadequate discharge planning, and inadequate information accompanying the patient regarding patient problems and conditions that warrant attention and treatment. On the receiving end, long-term care providers are often not well staffed or equipped to assess patient needs properly and comprehensively in order to avoid costly hospitalizations and complications, and to maximize patient well-being. This is especially problematic for near-acute patients who would benefit from a reasonable (but not excessive) assessment of care needs to determine rehabilitation potential and prognosis for purposes of care planning and treatment regimen. Too often are near-acute patients with rehabilitation potential admitted to nursing homes that retain such patients far longer than necessary, possibly bringing about a level of dependency in the patient that is totally inappropriate. At the extreme, this can result in a permanent nursing home stay—when proper assessment, care planning, and patient management would have resulted in discharge within several weeks to an independent living environment.

In Chapter 7, it was noted that Merrill and Somers (1989) speak of an "infrastructure" needed before we delve too deeply into the issue of how to comprehensively finance long-term care in the United States. This is a point well worth heeding. Until we know how to structure and integrate the various types of long-term care, as well as how to integrate long-term care and acute care, it may be premature to be discussing how much money we need to support a comprehensive long-term care delivery system—premature in the sense that we do not know precisely what it is that we are trying to integrate and, therefore, how it should be unified. The thoughts and suggestions contained in the remainder of this chapter are intended to shed some light on essential attributes of near-acute care, parameters that are vital to integrating near-acute care with existing care modalities, and steps to finalizing the best ways to do this. It is my opinion that better integration, carefully planned and structured, need not result in increased cost to our entire system. It will, in fact, result in either decreased cost or, even if we chose to invest more, increased cost effectiveness.

Rehabilitation Care and Maintenance Care Philosophies: A Difference to Emphasize

Many of us in the United States typically think of nursing homes as places where old people go to die. The real tragedy is that because we think this way, it happens more often than it should. It is true that many nursing homes serve but one type of resident—the chronically ill patient whose stay may be for a period of several years, possibly until death. It is also true that we have relatively few nursing homes that specialize exclusively in rehabilitating patients so that they can return to independent living settings. A reasonable number of nursing homes, in fact, care for both types of patients in the same facility.

Our research in swing-bed care has highlighted the pronounced differences that exist between rehabilitation care provided in a traditional chronic care setting versus a more therapeutic or rehabilitation setting. Most nursing homes that are equipped and staffed primarily to provide traditional or chronic long-term care are characterized by a philosophy of maintenance and palliation. It is important that residents who receive chronic care or maintenance care be treated with dignity and respect, ensuring an adequate quality of life. Many such patients must be maintained comfortably, making serious efforts to minimize the rate of functional loss or the occurrence of other physiological, cognitive, emotional, or medical problems. The philosophy that characterizes such care, however, is radically different from the philosophy that characterizes rehabilitation care for shorter-term patients, who should be encouraged to improve in functioning so that they can function independently upon discharge from the institution.

Our finding that swing-bed hospitals were considerably more successful at providing rehabilitation care and encouraging patients to be discharged to independent living is consistent with the philosophy that accompanies acute care. The typical philosophy in an acute care setting is curative in nature, with the general expectation that patients will improve after receiving hospital care and be discharged home. This philosophy carries over when long-term care is provided in swing beds,

resulting in higher discharge rates to independent living, less rehospitalization after discharge, and attainment of greater levels of independent
functioning for swing-bed patients than for rural nursing home patients,
even after taking into consideration differences in the types of patients
found in the two settings. On the other hand, nursing homes in rural
communities are better at providing maintenance care to chronically ill
patients whose stays are considerably longer than the two- to three-
week stays of patients rehabilitated in swing-bed hospitals. The substantially higher numbers of physician visits and the higher proportions of
skilled nurses in the acute care hospital setting, combined with a curative philosophy, render the provision of near-acute care both more natural and more successful in swing beds than in nursing homes. In general, the findings point to a need to consider the circumstances and care
modalities under which rehabilitation care and chronic care should be
provided.

Patient Needs, Types of Care, and Providers of Care

Geriatric assessment, in comprehensive form, refers to a thorough interdisciplinary team assessment of a geriatric patient's care needs. Such
assessments are typically conducted on an inpatient basis in the more
comprehensive geriatric assessment and treatment units—of which
there are relatively few in the United States. A typical assessment might
involve a number of cognitive, emotional, physiological, and functional
components, which, considered in conjunction with the patient's history and results from other diagnostic tests, form the basis for determining
the patient's care needs and prognosticating likely outcomes under a
specific treatment plan. A full-blown geriatric assessment, with a number of health care professionals in a relatively well-equipped environment, is neither possible nor practical for the vast majority of geriatric
patients in our country. Nor are the extensive services that go into such
an assessment necessarily cost-effective for all types of geriatric patients.
Nevertheless, common sense as well as research findings we have to
date would suggest that selected elements of geriatric assessment and
ensuing treatment probably form critical ingredients of near-acute care,
especially for patients with rehabilitation potential.

    While we still have great distances to travel in prognosticating
patient outcomes and determining rehabilitation potential, a reasonably
thorough assessment would seem to hold the key for significant improvements in providing near-acute care to patients with rehabilitation
potential. Once a care plan is established for such a patient, it is as
important to monitor and reassess patient status intermittently as it is to
follow through with the care program. It is entirely possible for a patient

initially judged to have moderate or minimal rehabilitation potential to make more significant strides toward rehabilitation than originally expected. We have seen this occur for both swing-bed patients and patients in other rehabilitation settings. Likewise, a patient with strong rehabilitation potential may not progress as rapidly because of complicating factors, such as respiratory problems that are not responding to treatment or a surgical wound that does not heal as expected. If a patient is an acute care patient prior to placement in near-acute care, discharge planning in the hospital is a critical first step in monitoring and managing care. The location to which the patient is discharged must have the capacity to provide services that are consistent with the *predischarge* assessment and care plan. It is at this point where hospitals and physicians often encounter problems. Not only are adequate predischarge assessments and good discharge planning too infrequent, but even in those cases where they might be adequately done, the preferred posthospital setting might not be available for the patient. Many hospitals and hospital staff throughout the country are encountering difficulties in properly placing near-acute patients.

Rarely is a consistent, comprehensive, and uniform approach or recording form established prior to hospital discharge that has clear and definitive requirements for specifying and updating the care plan in keeping with reassessments of the near-acute care patient's condition and care needs—particularly when discharged from hospital to nursing home. Rarely is a single individual designated who functions as a care coordinator throughout the episode of near-acute care; that is, only infrequently does one person serve as a continually present patient care advocate who interacts with all providers as needed to update and change the care plan with the frequency dictated by the patient's changing condition until the patient is discharged to independent living or the determination is made that the patient cannot be rehabilitated.

Much of this happens rather naturally, however, in the rural swing-bed environment: a patient discharged from acute care to long-term care remains in the same institution, in an acute care bed, with the same nursing staff, and with the physician continuing to visit far more frequently than we typically encounter in other long-term care environments. The hospital discharge planner, a nurse, or the swing-bed coordinator might play the role of care coordinator, typically working closely with physicians and nurses since acute care and near-acute long-term care are provided in the same acute care facility. The necessary coordination, transfer of records, monitoring of patient status, managing and updating the care plan in keeping with patient needs, and reassessments of patient status occur naturally. When a patient requires a diagnostic workup or medical services that might typically entail transferring a nursing home patient to a hospital for either inpatient or emergency care, it is often done in a swing-bed hospital without any such transfer. Equally important, the accompanying costs and trauma to the patient are avoided. Many of the essential ingredients of high-quality near-acute care are present and occur naturally.

Thus, near-acute cases are managed efficiently, not necessarily always with the same individual managing a given patient's care from start to finish, but typically with reasonably clear communication, transfer of records, and provider knowledge of the patient's acute care history and its ramifications for near-acute care and potential rehabilitation. Skilled nursing services are readily available. Multidisciplinary assessment and coordinated care management is the rule rather than the exception. At least one physician is involved in continually monitoring the patient and possibly changing the care plan on a frequent basis, far more frequently than is found in typical nursing homes. Services tend to be well integrated and reviewed. While underprovision or overprovision of certain types of services is of course possible, they are less likely because the multidisciplinary approach followed inherently contains its own system of checks and balances.

If a swing-bed long-term care patient is likely to be a chronic long-term care patient, he or she would probably be discharged from the facility after the acute stay unless some hope exists for rehabilitation, warranting at least a trial stay in the more therapeutic environment of the hospital. There are exceptions to this, of course, since a few swing-bed hospitals continue to provide more traditional long-term care. Some do so successfully, others not as well. By and large, however, the primary orientation of swing-bed hospitals has been directed toward near-acute care. Some swing-bed hospitals do not provide such care as well as others, but on average they seem to be doing a remarkable job. Nonetheless, at any given time, 20 to 40 percent of swing-bed patients may be awaiting placement in other more chronic care settings, such as nursing homes or residential care facilities. The exceptional performance on the part of swing-bed hospitals pertains not to these patients, but to the near-acute care patients.

The physician is often the forgotten provider in the long-term care field. In the first chapter, it was emphasized that the evolution of public sector reimbursement and regulatory policy in the long-term care field over the last 50 years was marked by the rather conspicuous absence of physician involvement. In fact, the manner in which we pay for and regulate physician involvement in the long-term care field today highlights the paucity of concern about, and failure to recognize, the significance of physician care for long-term care patients. This is exacerbated by the problem that medical education and physician practice are often but minimally involved with or oriented toward nursing home care and long-term care in general. It is my opinion that the primary reason why too few patients are properly rehabilitated and discharged from nursing homes to independent living arrangements rests with the inadequate involvement of physicians in long-term care, especially in caring for near-acute patients who have moderate or even poor rehabilitation potential (but who are judged to have some such potential). We give up on such patients too easily and too quickly.

Not to be forgotten as potentially important providers of care or influences on outcomes of care, are the patient and the patient's family. For some types of care, most notably home health care, the roles of the patient and the patient's family and home support system are often pivotal. Knowledge of self-care, compliance with a treatment regimen, and emotional support are all ingredients of a home care program. Thus, such "providers of care" cannot be overlooked in the rehabilitation process.

Reimbursement and Financing

As discussed in Chapter 7, during the past several years a number of proposals have been proffered on how to finance long-term care in the United States. Many of these suggestions have been well thought out in terms of financing mechanisms and approaches. Most are premised on the valid assumption that long-term care is seriously fragmented and poorly integrated; most are also premised on the assumption that we need considerably more money for long-term care in the United States. Understandably, however, most do not state definitively what it is that we are to integrate and, more importantly, precisely how we should integrate various types of long-term care with, for example, acute care and outpatient care.

Recently, we have also had suggestions and discussions on issues related to bundling long-term care services, even with acute care services in some instances, and paying for such services through some type of combined or capitated rate. Some of these have focused on the proposal that hospitals could broker long-term care. The basic idea is that the hospital, either as part of its DRG payment or through some other financing mechanism, should be paid for both acute care and long-term care. It would manage the long-term care received by patients after discharge from acute care, whether such care be in a hospital-based unit, a freestanding nursing home, or even a home care arrangement. On the surface, this is attractive from a financing perspective since it "black boxes" at least some types of long-term care at the end of an acute care stay. It has the theoretical attraction that accompanies various forms of capitation: payers can leave the decisions on precisely what types of care a patient ought to receive—and even the trade-offs associated with various types of care—to the provider by simply paying a preset amount for combined acute and long-term care (or for long-term care at the end of an acute stay). Unfortunately, however, these simplifying features that are attractive on conceptual grounds mask difficulties that might bring about significant problems in effectiveness and quality of care.

As suggested earlier, even the hospitals participating in our national swing-bed program in rural communities do not provide or manage chronic care and maintenance care very well relative to other long-term care providers. To have hospitals and hospital staff in charge of brokering such care on the grounds of financial or reimbursement considerations alone simply does not make much sense. On the other hand, hospitals and hospital staff appear to be able to provide and manage near-acute care well. To properly discuss a service-bundling or capitation approach, we have to be specific about the type of long-term care (e.g., near-acute rather than chronic/maintenance care) that lends itself to such arrangements. We might well be able to do a great deal more to improve the quality of near-acute care without infusing more total dollars into our health care system if acute care providers were to broker near-acute care—but not the full range of subacute long-term care, which includes chronic care and maintenance care. This might enable us to make significant inroads into improved quality and effectiveness of near-acute care, at least for patients who are discharged from hospitals requiring such care (recall that near-acute care patients need not be discharged from hospitals, although the vast majority of such patients are posthospital patients).

We Must Innovate to Gain a Return

Cost cannot be the overriding and exclusive consideration in exploring alternatives for innovation, especially in the near-acute care field. The success of the swing-bed program has taught us that while we might pay more on a per day basis for better integrated and more effective near-acute care, it can ultimately cost our total health care system less to provide such care because of the savings that can accrue from reduced hospitalization rates and reduced use of outpatient services. In several areas, we have probably been penny-wise and pound-foolish in not investigating certain types of health care innovations because, on the surface, they *might* cost more than seems apparent under the status quo. While demonstrations have been a normal accompaniment of the Medicare and Medicaid programs over their first 25 years, there is, at times, inappropriate resistance to endorsing and encouraging demonstrations because "demonstrations always result in expanding patient benefits and therefore spending more money." Sometimes this is the case. Other times it is not. In any event, the cost of demonstrations, evaluations, and research about extant programs (especially in view of their potential benefits) is truly inconsequential relative to new or continuing program costs under Medicare.

At a minimum, good demonstrations and accompanying evaluations shed light not only on how much a new type of (or approach to) care will cost, but also on the degree to which it will improve effectiveness and possibly enhance overall cost effectiveness. It makes no sense to bury our heads in the sand by not trying new approaches, or by not thoroughly evaluating them to determine whether their strengths outweigh their weaknesses. We have now come sufficiently far in our ability to design and structure demonstrations in the health care field, and to comprehensively evaluate them, so that they can be extremely beneficial undertakings. This was not always true, especially during the first 10 to 15 years after the Medicare program was implemented. It is now possible to capitalize on our experience and the methods that we have spent years fine-tuning. Equally important, we have many naturally occurring innovations initiated by providers or groups of providers. We can often learn a great deal by investigating and researching such programs with the range of available expertise and analytic methods.

We simply will not be able to solve our problems in the areas of financing, access, quality, and overall cost effectiveness unless we objectively and thoroughly analyze our present weaknesses and experiment with new approaches. Wholesale, sweeping changes that have not been well tested can be costly, dangerous, and highly inefficient. For example, as noble and well intended as our expansion of long-term care (and other) benefits was under the Medicare Catastrophic Coverage Act of 1988 were, no one really knew how well it would be received and how effective it would prove to be. The loss of time, money, and resources invested in passing this act and then repealing it was immense. A few well-planned demonstrations and evaluation programs would have probably paved the way for how to best structure the approach—and ensure more widespread acceptance of the recommended changes, if any. If we do not want to pay for some degree of experimentation and investigation, we will perforce innovate in big gulps. We may be lucky sometimes, but big losers in other instances. Yet, the cost of systematic and well–thought out innovation is minuscule, in fact truly negligible compared with the cost of being big losers even once, to say nothing of several times. Realistically, our political and legislative process, as well as the unpredictability of many societal needs, is such that we will never be able to totally avoid new but untested national initiatives and programs. When this occurs, we will simply have to continue to trust our luck. However, we should be as diligent as possible in our efforts to act on the merits of testing innovations before making large-scale changes.

EFFECTING HEALTH POLICY CHANGE
IN THE NEAR-ACUTE CARE FIELD

Overview

We desperately need a road map of how to change our health care system so that long-term care is well integrated with other types of health care. While such a road map is beyond the purview of this book, a starting point and an initial road to travel are proposed. The starting point for policy change directed toward better integrating acute and long-term care should be improved near-acute care for patients judged to have some potential for rehabilitation. The phrase "potential for re-habilitation" here means only that there is a modest chance to rehabili-tate, not necessarily that the patient has strong rehabilitation potential (although it clearly includes such patients).

To begin with near-acute care patients who have at least some rehabilitation potential has several advantages. First, such patients are typically discharged from acute care to long-term care. We have accumu-lated a substantial knowledge base over the past ten years regarding how to integrate acute care and long-term care cost-effectively for these specific types of patients. Second, elderly near-acute care patients are typically among the patients who are eligible for the Medicare SNF benefit. The influence that the Medicare program can exert on providers through reimbursement and administrative incentives is powerful. Modest changes in this benefit by Medicare for such patients can there-fore serve as the catalyst or change agent in this regard. Third, we currently have serious problems in near-acute care that result in un-necessarily high expense and ineffectiveness from the perspectives of both cost and quality of care. Since we now have the requisite knowl-edge at our disposal on how to solve such problems, our only challenge is to determine which (or what blend) of several competing alternatives represents the optimal way to solve these problems.

Fourth, because of its proximity to acute care, near-acute care repre-sents an appropriate springboard or transition point for improved inte-gration between long-term care and acute hospital care (and, in some ways, outpatient/physician care). Near-acute long-term care for patients with rehabilitation potential is a reasonably well-circumscribed modality of long-term care that can be strongly influenced through Medicare initiatives. At the same time, it can be viewed as the center of a series of concentric circles of types of long-term care that we can progressively integrate more effectively with other types of health care through policy initiatives. Through progressive change starting with near-acute care, we can enhance our ability to coordinate care from the viewpoints of quality maximization and cost control. Thus, we can expand our purview of improved integration to progressively larger targeted groups of patients and patient care if we begin with near-acute patients.

The importance of near-acute care was established in earlier chapters. Hospital discharge represents a key entry point to the long-term care system for a significant proportion of long-term care patients. Further, analyses of health service utilization patterns of long-term care patients over time demonstrate that hospital admission is often the reason for discharge from long-term care settings—owing to complications, decline in health status, or serious exacerbations of chronic care problems that, if treated effectively in long-term care settings, might not require hospitalization. The likelihood that an elderly patient receiving care in our long-term care system will be a near-acute care patient over a one- to two-year period is substantial. Thus, by seeking to improve near-acute care, we will begin to structure the critical ingredients of care integration and coordination for a large number of patients in our long-term care delivery system. If we then expand our purview to near-acute care patients with little or no rehabilitation potential in our next concentric ring, we will be reaching a large majority of all long-term care patients.

We know that the more essential features of near-acute care include the following:

1. reasonably thorough assessment of the patient's rehabilitation potential, general prognosis, and ensuing care needs
2. provision of services in accord with a well-defined and monitored care plan coordinated preferably by a single individual from the time before hospital discharge (if hospitalization was involved) through discharge from near-acute care
3. reasonably frequent monitoring of the care plan and reassessment of patient status to modify the care plan
4. increased physician involvement and attentiveness
5. provision of therapeutic, skilled nursing and, if appropriate, social services in keeping with the total care needs (medical, functional, behavioral, cognitive, and emotional) of the patient

It would appear that a thorough initial assessment to screen most Medicare SNF patients to determine whether they qualify as near-acute care patients with at least some rehabilitation potential would be an important initial service. Thereafter, if the patient is determined to qualify, additional assessment (for some types of patients) beyond this first screening would be appropriate to determine the care plan.

Implementing a demonstration program or programs that incorporate variations on the above themes appears warranted. This could be done using urban swing-bed hospitals, for which demonstration authority exists. Nonetheless, urban swing-bed hospitals have never been tested as a means to address our near-acute care problems. A demonstration program could also involve Medicare-certified skilled nursing facilities (both hospital-based and freestanding) as well as both outpatient geriatric units and home health agencies as the organizational vehicles for near-acute care. We must be aware that the organizational base during an episode of near-acute care can change, for example, from a hospital swing-bed to a SNF and even to home care. Variations on the types of individuals responsible for coordinating care over the entire episode of near-acute care could be incorporated into such a demonstration program. Physicians or physician designees and nurse practitioners/nurse clinicians should be considered for the care coordinator role. Hospital staff nurses or swing-bed coordinators should also be considered for this role. In addition, since a number of innovations are under way that have been initiated by providers, a serious assessment of the cost effectiveness of emerging provider-initiated approaches to near-acute care would be beneficial.

Once a satisfactory definition of near-acute care patients with rehabilitation potential is developed, a combined demonstration and research program can be implemented to determine the most cost-effective modalities and combinations of providers for integrating near-acute care with other types of health care. In fact, it would probably be possible to use a general definition of near-acute care in such a program, with the objective of refining it as a result of evaluating the program. As mentioned, it is no longer a question of whether such care can be cost-effectively integrated, since we have now witnessed this occurring in several settings. Rather, our highly feasible task is to assess which are the best types of provider combinations, service combinations, and treatment approaches for different types of near-acute care patients. We would then be ready, within a few years, possibly three to five years, to change the Medicare SNF benefit to offer a near-acute care benefit to specific types of SNF patients. The demonstration programs, and very likely the final policy changes, should, at a minimum, incorporate Medicare coverage for screening and assessment services for near-acute care patients with rehabilitation potential, periodic reassessment and coordination services over a 7- to 45-day stay in near-acute care, and increased physician visits. Based on our experiences to date, we would expect the cost of the services to be offset by decreased hospitalization and reduced use of other institutional and noninstitutional long-term care after discharge from near-acute care.

Broad Goals

In all, to begin to better integrate and coordinate long-term care and other types of health care in the United States we should

— start with a concerted effort to improve the quality and cost effectiveness of near-acute long-term care;

— take advantage of the existing supply of health care providers by offering them incentives to integrate services for near-acute patients; and

— adopt a clear cost-effectiveness orientation in judging the success of alternative approaches to near-acute care—that is, use patient outcomes compared with the cost of care to assess which options and care modalities are most successful.

The remainder of the discussion in this section deals first with issues to consider in the context of attaining the above goals, and then with steps that appear essential to actually change our present system so that we might attain the above three goals.

Short-Term Recommendations for Near-Acute Care

General Objective. In striving for a system of acute care, postacute care, and long-term care that is better integrated than our present system, the dominant theme of this integration should be improved patient outcomes. If our initial focus is on near-acute care for patients with rehabilitation potential, it is likely that we can accomplish this objective without increasing the cost of health care in the United States.

Definition of Near-Acute Care. We must define precisely what we mean by near-acute care so that it can be well circumscribed for reimbursement and regulatory purposes. From the perspective of good patient care, there is often an artificiality to such definitions, yet the nature of our health care system dictates this as a necessity. The key parameters of such a definition would appear to be the extent of physician services, skilled nursing services, rehabilitation potential, assessment and reassessment, and care coordination required by the patient. As a general starting point, but with no pretense made that this is a rigorous definition for reimbursement purposes, near-acute patients with rehabilitation potential can be defined as patients who would benefit substantially (e.g., have at least a 20 percent likelihood of being discharged to an independent living environment from either institutional care, outpatient care, or home care) from

1. up to four physician visits per week;
2. skilled nursing or therapeutic services of at least seven hours per week;
3. weekly reassessments of physiologic, functional, cognitive, and emotional needs by a team consisting at least of a physician and skilled nurse, possibly augmented by a physical therapist, social worker, or other disciplines depending on patient needs; and
4. a single coordinator of care responsible for monitoring patient status and the patient's care plan over the near-acute care episode,

where discharge to independent living is expected to occur within 45 days of admission to near-acute care in an institutional or noninstitutional setting.

The above definition should be scrutinized, reviewed, and refined as appropriate from the perspective of the expected volume and types of services specified. In addition, patient conditions and characteristics should be included. For example, without doubt orthopedic conditions such as certain types of fractures (e.g., hip fracture) that require surgical procedures, various types of other postsurgical patients, and certain types of CVAs or stroke patients would be included. Further, specific risk factors or covariates that substantially lessen rehabilitation potential for independent living, such as serious cognitive impairments, neurological disorders, and chronic functional problems that render a patient dependent on institutional care, should be taken into consideration. It would appear necessary for demonstration and research purposes only to illustrate the types of conditions and risk factors that delineate near-acute care with rehabilitation potential from other types of long-term care. Provider and clinical judgment could be used in demonstration and research programs, with research on the resultant practices and analyses providing the basis for a more specific operational delineation of near-acute care patients that would be incorporated into a national policy change under Medicare.

Increased Physician Involvement in Near-Acute Care. To facilitate improved medical care, assessment and reassessment of patient condition, care planning and management, and intermittent changes in care planning and management, it is imperative to increase the involvement of physicians in near-acute care. Our experiences to date with increased physician involvement for near-acute care patients strongly suggest that it is not only in the interest of patients, but in the long run it can reduce costs for such patients and is therefore in the best interest of payers. As recommended earlier, payment for more frequent physician visits to near-acute care patients appears warranted from the perspectives of both quality and the total cost of care.

Permitting Multiple Provider Settings for Near-Acute Care. Depending on a patient's condition, circumstances, community resources, and the availability of different types of provider settings in a given location, near-acute care can feasibly be provided in or through hospital swing beds, hospital-based nursing homes, freestanding nursing homes, geriatric outpatient clinics, and home health care programs. The successes in cost-effectively providing near-acute care have occurred largely in institutional settings to date. However, assuming the patient is neither bed-bound nor immobile, there is at least some reason to believe that a well-coordinated approach to near-acute care could be effective in noninstitutional or outpatient/day-care settings as well. It would be appropriate to proceed slowly (e.g., on a more limited demonstration basis, or by evaluating extant programs that provide coordinated near-acute care) with noninstitutional care.

Improved Assessment and Reassessment. We should approximate, but not totally replicate, geriatric assessment as performed in the more comprehensive geriatric assessment and treatment units at the present time. It does not appear that an extremely comprehensive assessment of all patients as a matter of routine is necessary. Rather, for near-acute care patients with rehabilitation potential, an assessment that focuses on key patient conditions and needs, involving multidisciplinary input, should suffice. Periodic reassessments, targeted on patient needs identified in the care plan resulting from the first assessment, should be conducted, possibly weekly or biweekly since the targeted patients will be judged to have rehabilitation potential.

As mentioned, the first assessment could occur in two stages. The first stage would be a screen to determine whether the patient can be classified as a near-acute care patient with moderate rehabilitation potential. The second would be to develop the care plan for eligible patients. Eligibility for the near-acute care benefit should be well defined to eliminate subjectivity and minimize the tendency to fit many more types of patients into the category than belong.

Increased Coordination of Near-Acute Care. Beginning with the initial assessment to determine whether a patient qualifies for near-acute care, a specific qualified individual, who might be termed the near-acute care coordinator for the patient, should be assigned to monitor patient status and patient care throughout the duration of the patient's stay in a near-acute care setting or settings. If, for example, the initial assessment were done in a hospital setting, the care coordinator might be a hospital-assigned staff member with qualifications for monitoring such care. If the initial assessment were done in a nursing home setting, an analogous qualified nursing home staff member might be assigned this responsibility. It might be possible and appropriate to assign a qualified individual from outside the organization to be involved in the initial assessment and to monitor patient status, care provided, and changes in care plans and reassessments over the course of the patient's stay in near-acute care. Ideally, this individual would not only be responsible for monitoring care, but should be an active participant in assessment, reassessment, and care planning.

The qualifications of the near-acute care coordinator are especially important. For certain types of case management and channeling programs that have existed for over a decade, the case manager has often been a social worker or someone trained more strongly in the areas of social and emotional care than medical or skilled nursing care. This may be desirable for chronic care patients whose predominant needs are often in these areas or in areas that require mostly support and functional care, but the needs of near-acute patients are dominated by requirements related to medical, skilled nursing, and therapeutic care. As a result, the near-acute care coordinator should be skilled and knowledgeable in these areas, with the ability to communicate with other disciplines about behavioral, social, and emotional needs of near-acute care patients. Thus, the model proposed for near-acute care is radically different from case management and channeling for more chronic care patients. In fact, case management has encountered mixed success, at times bordering on failure, in these areas. Some have conjectured it is because of the breadth of needs that often characterize chronic care patients with cognitive, social, or emotional problems; others conjecture that insufficient attention was paid to the need for medical and skilled nursing services by case managers who were not sufficiently knowledgeable in these areas; and still others contend that adequate services were not available to manage care correctly. In any event, more traditional case management for chronic care patients and care coordination for near-acute care patients as recommended here are radically different.

Improved Skilled Nursing Involvement in Near-Acute Care. As emphasized in earlier chapters, a rehabilitative/restorative philosophy should characterize near-acute care for patients with rehabilitation potential. In this regard, skilled nurses, who are likely to be the dominant providers of care to such patients, should be continually involved in monitoring patient status and providing or directly supervising all nursing care. If nurses aides or their equivalents are involved in the provision of care, they should be trained and managed in keeping with a curative or therapeutic philosophy of care consistent with encouraging patient independence. We must bear in mind that this philosophy is the antithesis of fostering patient dependence on the part of care providers, something that understandably occurs very frequently in providing support services to chronically ill long-term care patients in many nursing homes.

Initial Focus on Discharge to Independent Living. The recommendation to focus initially on near-acute care patients with rehabilitation potential perforce requires that we work toward discharging such patients to an independent living environment. To qualify for near-acute care of this type, it must be anticipated that a patient has at least a reasonable chance of living independently, where independent living must also take into consideration the patient's home environment. A patient with family support at home may not require as high a degree of independent living skills as a patient who has no family or outside support at home. If it is highly unlikely that an individual could be discharged to an independent living setting (including a residential care institution), then the initial focus on near-acute care with rehabilitation potential would preclude such a patient from qualifying for this benefit. Nonetheless, subsequent broadening of the benefit could include near-acute care for patients with little or no rehabilitation potential. Concurrent research and policy analysis should therefore be conducted on how to best integrate and coordinate such care with other types of health care.

Reimbursement Changes. The most critical additional features of near-acute care specified above—for which we do not presently pay—are increased physician care, assessment and reassessment services, and improved care coordination. Even under a demonstration program, some form of Medicare reimbursement changes would be necessary to compensate providers for such care. The manner in which such reimbursement changes or policies might be structured by Medicare (and Medicaid) would depend on the preferred approach by these two public payers. It is likely that Medicare payment to physicians for near-acute care would continue to go through Medicare Part B, that the assessment and reassessment services could be covered through fee-for-service reimbursement to the organizational provider that has overall responsibility for the assessment and reassessment services, and that the care coordinator services could also be covered through increased reimbursement to the organizational entity that has responsibility for care coordination. As an alternative, it would be possible for such an organizational entity to receive a lump-sum payment or partial payments for care coordination and the purchase of physician and assessment/reassessment services.

Uniqueness of Long-Term Care, Need for Physician Involvement, and Differences between Rehabilitation and Maintenance Care. However we decide to provide, regulate, and pay for near-acute care, we must remember that long-term care is far different from acute care. Although near-acute care is closer to hospital care than other types of long-term care, it still is not the same as acute or hospital care. First, considerably longer average stays, far less ability to rely on diagnosis as a determinant of resource requirements and cost of care, and a greater need to be aware of and respond to the nonmedical needs of patients—all these place near-acute care in the domain of long-term care. We are not yet able to develop a combined payment system for acute care and near-acute care so that Medicare might employ a combined payment, in the form of an extended DRG payment, for a combined acute/near-acute episode of care, although this may be feasible in the long run. Second, as mentioned several times, it is important to emphasize that physician involvement in the long-term care field in general, and in near-acute care in particular, remains inadequate. Third, it is difficult in any provider setting to mix rehabilitation care and maintenance care. While it is certainly possible to do so—and some nursing homes are effectively doing this—we should assess whether those nursing homes that provide relatively small amounts of rehabilitation care, especially to Medicare patients, and large amounts of maintenance care to longer-stay patients are sufficiently well oriented, in terms of a rehabilitation philosophy, to mix both types of care.

Investigating the Most Effective Options to Providing Near-Acute Long-Term Services and Settings. In addition to a demonstration program to precisely test the aforementioned approaches and options, we should research the several different approaches we currently have in place to provide near-acute long-term care. Some of these approaches might not be possible on a national scale either because of the unusually intense nature of services provided (and therefore the cost of such services), or because they do not adequately target patients for whom they are cost-effective. Nonetheless, they warrant a thorough and well-designed study to assess whether they might be cost-effective on a national level. Equally important, concurrently assessing the efficacy of different types of services and therapy programs would be possible and beneficial in the context of examining different provider settings.

Longer-Run Goals and Recommendations for Near-Acute Care

Expanded Scope of Change. As we learn more about how to provide and pay for near-acute care for patients with rehabilitation potential, we should consider how to provide and pay for such care to patients who do not have rehabilitation potential. It may be that the current methods of providing SNF care are sufficient. Enhanced care coordination for some types of SNF patients may be possible under our current payment approach simply by pointing out what is necessary and how it can be done under our current reimbursement practices. This would warrant further analysis, as well as a more comprehensive examination of how we pay for postacute care in general.

Improved Methods to Assess Rehabilitation Potential and to Prognosticate. We presently rely strongly on provider judgment to determine the extent to which a patient can be rehabilitated. Provider judgment implicitly but subjectively takes into consideration a number of factors: for example, patient status, history, care provided in the past, and signs and symptoms. Yet, we have done relatively little research (using longitudinal data) into predicting what outcomes might occur with relatively optimal rehabilitation care as a function of patient condition, risk factors, and other circumstances. This would be a highly fruitful area for research not only for the sake of improving near-acute care, but also for acute and long-term care patients in general.

Improved Methods to Monitor Outcomes. The most important way to assess the effectiveness of near-acute care is in terms of what happens to the patient. While discharge to independent living, with no or relatively minor problems for a reasonable period of time thereafter, is the outcome of choice, several other types of outcomes should be monitored. For example, improvement in the areas of functional abilities, wound healing, absence of infection, diminution of postsurgical depression, stabilization of blood pressure, and improved ability to carry out instrumental activities of daily living should be monitored for different types of patients. Analogously, hospitalizations and rehospitalizations should be examined for appropriateness or inappropriateness. Risk factors or covariates that can influence such outcomes need to be reasonably well specified and, if possible, standards established so that we can assess whether outcomes are attained with sufficient consistency by providers of near-acute care.

Estimation of the Cost of Near-Acute Care. An episode of near-acute care is likely to last anywhere from 7 to 45 days. We need to determine the cost of such care for different types of patients so that we might revise and refine our approach to reimbursement for near-acute care patients over time. It is conceivable that we can divide near-acute care patient types into a number of groups as we have done with DRGs in the hospital field. In this regard, the feasibility of paying for an episode of near-acute care according to patient types should be investigated and, if appropriate, implemented. It is not presently possible to combine near-acute case-mix groups with DRGs for hospital care. However, bundling near-acute care services by type of near-acute care patient for reimbursement purposes would represent a significant step forward in cost-effective reimbursement for near-acute care that encourages coordinated and well-managed care.

Study and Selection of Appropriate Reimbursement Methods. Over the course of time, as we gain experience with the provision of near-acute care, it is highly likely that a single approach to paying for such care under Medicare, at least, would emerge. In view of information that we have at our disposal presently, our goal might most appropriately be reimbursement per episode, rather than per day, of near-acute care. Such an approach would require developing a near-acute care patient grouping scheme, where reimbursement per episode might vary as a function of patient types (mentioned above). This could be implemented on a demonstration basis in order to estimate cost as well as refine patient groupings, and to assess the quality of care relative to cost.

Capitalizing on Existing Provider Capacity. Our current capacity to provide near-acute care is substantial. This is not to say, however, that we have structured and integrated our health care system to provide such care well. We have a large number of empty hospital beds throughout the country that could be used as swing beds to provide many types of institutional near-acute care. This is certainly the case in urban hospitals where a swing-bed demonstration has never been attempted. A number of nursing homes have a strong and well-established rehabilitation orientation that can be used to provide near-acute care, with the added ingredients, at least in many instances, of increased physician care, better and more frequent assessments, and a more coordinated approach to such care. It is likely that physicians would become more integrally involved in such care if reimbursement incentives were offered to do so. In reorienting, but not rebuilding, our current provider system, we must bear in mind that providers of care do best what comes naturally. To attempt to reorient chronic care facilities to provide near-acute care to rehabilitation patients, for example, would be foolish and unnecessarily costly. To build new freestanding nursing homes that would specialize in this type of care also would appear to be inefficient and cost-ineffective.

Flexible Regulation. As we move forward with improved patient care and reimbursement methods for near-acute care, it will be necessary to change our approaches to certification, accreditation, quality assurance, and utilization review for such care. As was done with the swing-bed program in its demonstration stages, and even in its initial stages as a national program, the spirit of our regulatory approach should be consistent with our efforts to innovate. It is to be expected that our regulatory approach should unfold as our approach to near-acute care unfolds. Thus, regulators and providers alike should expect to go through an educational process.

CONCLUDING REMARK

We have learned a great deal from a number of health policy developments over the past 20 years. One of these, the evolution of swing-bed care, has taught us two important lessons. First, health policy can be developed in a reasonably rational manner by testing sound proposals to improve the cost effectiveness of care through demonstration projects and research. The results of such research can be used to shape and implement a revised or new policy that embodies an optimal approach to providing such care. Even when implementing a new national program, we can benefit further from an evolution-shaping model program involving selected providers that are given incentives to implement the new national program sooner and possibly more comprehensively than others. Other providers, and even payers and regulators, can benefit from the initial experience gained from the model program put in place at the outset of a national program.

Second, the swing-bed approach has helped us recognize the strong need for, and the essential attributes of, near-acute care. No formula-like approach to providing near-acute care was advocated in this book because it appears that several different approaches may be cost-effective. By taking advantage of existing provider capacity in a research and demonstration program to determine the optimal blend and roles of different providers known to be effective in the near-acute care field, we may well learn how to structure and implement a new national policy in this area in the not too distant future.

CHAPTER 8 SUMMARY

Our experience with the evolution of hospital swing beds has indicated that providers of health care can adapt remarkably well to innovation if the new approach capitalizes on the strengths and experience of the provider. A wide array of individuals expressed well-founded and serious doubts that long-term care could be cost-effectively provided in hospital beds used for both acute care and long-term care. As HCFA's experimentation with this innovation progressed, however, it became apparent that the vast majority of hospitals had successfully implemented the swing-bed approach by focusing on near-acute care and providing chronic or traditional long-term care only as necessary until other settings were available for the traditional long-term care patients. While there were some exceptions to this, the typical swing-bed hospital has proven to be an unusually effective provider of "short-term long-term care" because it is able to take advantage of its acute care orientation. This "naturalness phenomenon" very likely can be generalized to other care settings and innovations. We must bear in mind, that just as swing-bed hospitals are not oriented to providing maintenance or chronic care to long-term care patients, providers in general are unlikely to successfully implement innovations that are either antithetical to or radically different from their standard orientation to providing care. Rechanneling or redirecting an already existing strength or orientation of a provider, however, can yield considerable benefits.

The case of hospital swing beds substantiates our ability to test and refine health policy initiatives through demonstrations, evaluation, and research. When properly structured and objectively assessed, demonstrations, or even naturally occurring experiments initiated by providers, can yield high payoffs in shaping health policy at minimal expense. We are particularly likely to avoid the extremely high cost of starting and then repealing national programs (such as happened under the Medicare Catastrophic Coverage Act of 1988) if we are more diligent about testing the effectiveness of and receptivity to health services innovations before implementing them on a widespread basis. Equally important, we are more likely to design and discover better ways to provide health services by first testing new approaches.

The Robert Wood Johnson Foundation's (RWJF) model swing-bed program, implemented at the outset of the national program in the early 1980s, has further shown us that considerable benefit can accrue by encouraging a relatively small group of providers to implement programmatic change more rapidly at the outset of a new national initiative. Other providers can subsequently learn from the early experiences of the first wave of model providers. As mentioned in earlier chapters, the implementation of the national swing-bed program was relatively trouble-free. The hundreds of new hospitals, and even regulator agencies and payer-related programs, that began to participate in the mid-1980s benefited from the solutions to problems that had been worked through by, or on behalf of, the model hospitals that implemented swing-bed care in the early 1980s under the RWJF evolution-shaping demonstration.

In incrementally shaping health policy through demonstrations and research, two broad types of impediments are unavoidable. First, providers will frequently resist innovation, especially when it is accompanied by reimbursement or regulatory change. Such resistance is also likely when it is perceived that an increased level or volume of care is required under a new initiative without a commensurate change in reimbursement. Second, bureaucratic resistance to change within the context of administering our predominant public sector health care programs, Medicare and Medicaid, is to be expected. Health policy change, or even testing health policy change, frequently requires adapting regulatory or reimbursement practices. A bureaucracy structured to pay and regulate providers of care in a certain way is unlikely to alter its procedures efficiently, depending on the nature of the change required. Those involved in innovation must expect such resistance, view it as natural, and expect to spend time overcoming it. A number of reasons why an innovation should not be tried are commonly put forth under the guise of arguments that, for example, the innovation might be too costly or will result in only small changes that will not solve adequately large problems. Often, however, these reasons have their real basis in the inertia of and familiarity with the status quo that bring about provider or bureaucratic resistance to change.

In improving the manner in which we provide near-acute care, we should adopt several guiding principles. Near-acute care is a pivotal point on the spectrum of care that includes hospital care and long-term care. The extent to which we systematically integrate near-acute care into our health care system over the next five to ten years will be a barometer of how well we ultimately will be able to improve our methods for integrating acute care, long-term care, physician/outpatient care, and a variety of other types of care. It represents a relatively unique type of care that crosses a number of boundary points in the traditional but somewhat fragmented approach to health care in our fee-for-service system in the United States. By judiciously designing an infrastructure through reimbursement policy, regulation, market forces, and an awareness of the essential ingredients of near-acute care, we should be able to build a well-coordinated approach to such care. This approach should encourage considerably more cohesiveness and collaboration among a variety of care providers, including hospitals, nursing homes, rehabilitation units, physicians, home health agencies, skilled nurses, therapists, and social workers. If this can be accomplished within the domain of near-acute care, the potential for expansion and adaption into other areas of integration of health care services should be significant. This is not to say that we have a totally fragmented system at the present time. Rather, our health care system is far from cost-effective in view of what we are investing.

In implementing change in the long-term care field, and in near-acute care in particular, the difference between rehabilitation care and maintenance care is important. We must clearly address which environments are most appropriate for providing these two types of care. Equally important, the results of the swing-bed experience raise the question of whether traditional nursing homes that provide predominantly maintenance care should even be allowed to provide rehabilitation care to but a few patients at any given time. Analogously, providers that specialize predominantly in rehabilitation care or short-term long-term care should very likely be discouraged from providing maintenance care except on an interim basis until an appropriate setting becomes available.

Three of the most critical services to successfully providing high-quality near-acute care are assessment and reassessment of patient care needs, physician care, and a well-coordinated approach to monitoring and changing the care plan throughout the near-acute stay. While geriatric assessment programs have pointed to a number of desirable features of comprehensive patient assessment, we must be parsimonious in the manner in which we assess near-acute care patients because of our limited resources. The manner in which we pay for care coordination is important. For example, hospitals might be able to effectively broker near-acute care, but it is doubtful that they would be able to broker or effectively coordinate chronic or more traditional long-term care if paid a lump sum for doing so. In general, since we are aware of the essential factors that constitute good near-acute care, it remains to assess the most appropriate ways to integrate and provide such care; that is, it remains to determine the most appropriate provider settings for such care and the ways to achieve the greatest degree of integration.

Progress made during the 1970s, and particularly during the 1980s, has now shed considerable light on what is involved in effectively providing near-acute care. Before implementing a national policy change, very likely through a change in Medicare reimbursement for near-acute care patients, it would appear wise to test and assess different models for providing, coordinating, and paying for near-acute care. A combined demonstration/research program would necessarily have to begin with a definition of near-acute care and perhaps focus on near-acute care patients with rehabilitation potential, since the successes encountered thus far deal predominantly with these types of patients. To concentrate initially on such patients has the advantages of (1) starting with a clear vision of the types of patients for whom we will integrate acute and long-term care, (2) bringing the potential influence of Medicare reimbursement to bear as a powerful change agent, since a large majority of near-acute care patients are Medicare patients, (3) addressing a serious problem in our health care system today, and (4) providing a springboard to integration in other areas. Our initial goal should be to increase the quality and cost effectiveness of near-acute care, using the existing supply of providers (without necessarily creating a new type of specialty institution or discipline), and to judge the success of our various approaches on the basis of cost effectiveness and outcomes. A proposed starting point in defining near-acute care was given in this chapter. This definition was but a starting point since it was expressed in terms of required numbers of physician visits, skilled nursing and therapy services, frequency of assessments and reassessments, and care coordination. The definition was deliberately intended to be nonprescriptive, since the Medicare program is in a position to further refine it as a function of patient conditions and through a research and demonstration approach.

The ideal demonstration/research program would entail experimentation with increased physician involvement, multiple provider settings (including urban swing beds), improved assessment and reassessment methods, enhanced care coordination, various service regimens, and different experimental approaches to reimbursement. At one extreme, our current fee-for-service approaches can be implemented under a model that allows for more care coordination and increased physician and assessment services. At the other extreme, near-acute care can be brokered by an institutional or noninstitutional provider who receives a lump-sum payment for the provision of near-acute care that the provider is expected to coordinate by brokering services and paying for such care in accord with patient needs.

In analyzing how to provide near-acute care under Medicare, we must recognize that near-acute care is truly a type of long-term care. As such, it involves longer stays and different care needs than acute care. We cannot forecast long-term care needs exclusively on the basis of diagnoses and other attributes that forecast acute care needs reasonably well; therefore, we are not presently able to effectively and equitably pay hospitals prospectively for acute care and long-term care in the form of a single payment. We may be in a position in the relatively near future to structure a per case payment approach for patients at the outset of their near-acute stay, perhaps as part of a demonstration and research program. Some innovative programs for near-acute care exist in the context of health maintenance organizations (HMOs), however. Since capitation of the form practiced by HMOs represents the most extreme form of bundling, such programs warrant serious research from the perspectives of cost and quality.

As we finalize our approach to near-acute care, it is imperative that we continue to improve our methods to assess rehabilitation potential and predict patient outcomes as a function of patient conditions and treatment approaches. It is especially important that we identify risk factors and case-mix variables that distinguish between different resource needs, treatments, and likely outcomes for near-acute care patients. This will help in structuring reimbursement, quality assurance, and most importantly, cost-effective near-acute care. As we improve our methods to monitor outcomes for near-acute care patients, a more systematic approach to assuring the quality of this type of long-term care is likely to emerge. This will further assist in integrating different types of health care under the Medicare program. In studying and selecting the best reimbursement methods for near-acute care, our final determinations must, above all, be based on attaining the best possible outcomes for individual patients in view of what we can afford to pay for such care.

Bibliography

Achenbaum, W. 1978. *Old Age in the New Land.* Baltimore, MD: The Johns Hopkins University Press.

AFL-CIO. 1977. *Nursing Homes and the Nation's Elderly: America's Nursing Homes Profit in Human Misery.* Executive Council Statement and Report. Bal Harbour, FL.

American Bar Association. 1986. *The "Black Box" of Home Care Quality.* Presented by the chairman of the U.S. House Select Committee on Aging, Comm. Pub. No. 99-753, 99th Cong., 2d sess. Washington, D.C., August.

American Hospital Association (AHA). 1979a. *Status of the "Swing-Bed" Concept in the House and Senate.* Washington, D.C.: American Hospital Association.

————. 1979b. "Status of the 'Swing-Bed' Provision in the House and Senate." *Small and Rural Hospital Report,* November–December. Chicago, IL: American Hospital Association.

————. 1982. *Hospitals* 56(22).

————. 1989. "Transitional Care." *American Hospital Association, Section for Metropolitan Hospitals.* Chicago, IL.

Applegate, W., J. Blass, and T. Williams. 1990. "Review Article: Instruments for the Functional Assessment of Older Patients." *New England Journal of Medicine* 322(17):1207–13.

Avorn, J., and E. Langer. 1982. "Induced Disability in Nursing Home Patients: A Controlled Trial." *Journal of the American Geriatrics Society* 30(6):397–400.

Ball, R. 1990. "Public-Private Solution to Protection against the Cost of Long-Term Care." *Journal of the American Geriatrics Society* 38:156–63.

Beresford, L. 1990. "The Hospital Role in Post-Discharge Planning." *Medicine and Health: Perspectives* 44(9).

Bernstein, L. 1989. "Letters to the Editor: Functional Assessment in the Office." *Journal of the American Geriatrics Society* 37(5):490.

Bowlyow, J. 1990. "Acute and Long-Term Care Linkages: A Literature Review." *Medical Care Review* 47(1):75–103.

Brody, E. 1986. "The Role of the Family in Nursing Homes: Implications for Research and Public Policy." In *Mental Illness in Nursing Homes: Agenda for Research,* edited by M. Harper and B. Lebowitz. Rockville, MD: National Institute for Mental Health.

Brody, E., and S. Brody. 1989. "The Informal System of Health Care." In *Caring for the Elderly: Reshaping Health Policy,* edited by C. Eisendorfer, D. Kessler, and A. Spectors. Baltimore, MD: The Johns Hopkins University Press.

Buchanan, J., R. L. Kane, J. Garrard, R. Bell, C. Witsberger, A. Rosenfeld, C. Skay, and D. Gifford. 1989. *Results from the Evaluation of the Massachusetts Nursing Home Connection Program* (JR-01). Santa Monica, CA: The RAND Corporation.

Butler, R., and K. Hyer. 1989. "Reimbursement Reform for the Frail Elderly." *Journal of the American Geriatrics Society* 37(11):1097–98.

Carter, G., and P. Ginsburg. 1985. *The Medicare Case Mix Increase: Medical Practice Changes, Aging, and DRG Creep.* Prepared for Health Care Financing Administration, Cooperative Agreement No. 15-C-98489/9-01. Santa Monica, CA: The RAND Corporation.

Chekryn, J., and L. Roos. 1979. "Auditing the Process of Care in a New Geriatric Unit." *Journal of the American Geriatrics Society* 27(3):107–11.

Cohen, H., and J. Feussner. 1989. "Comprehensive Geriatric Assessment: Mission Not Yet Accomplished." *Journal of Gerontology* 44(6):M175–77.

Conklin, J., and R. Houchens. 1987. *PPS Impact on Mortality Rates: Adjustments for Case-Mix Severity.* Final Report: HCFA Contract No. 500-85-0015, 6 October.

Coward, R., and S. Cutler. 1989. "Informal and Formal Health Care Systems for the Rural Elderly." *Health Services Research* 23(6):785–806.

DeFriese, G., and T. Ricketts. 1989. "Primary Health Care in Rural Areas: An Agenda for Research." *Health Services Research* 23(6):931–74.

DeMaria, L. 1989. "Outpatient Geriatric Assessment." *Journal of the American Geriatrics Society* 37(11):1101–2.

DesHarnais, S., E. Kobrinski, J. Chesney, M. Long, R. Ament, and S. Fleming. 1987. "The Early Effects of the Prospective Payment System on Inpatient Utilization and the Quality of Care." *Inquiry* 24(1):7–16.

Dobrof, R., and E. Litwak. 1977. *Maintenance of Family Ties of Long-Term Care Patients: Theory and Guide to Practice.* Washington, D.C.: U.S. Government Printing Office.

Donabedian, A. 1980. *Explorations in Quality Assessment and Monitoring. Vol. 1: The Definition of Quality and Approaches to Its Assessment.* Ann Arbor, MI: Health Administration Press.

———. 1982. *Explorations in Quality Assessment and Monitoring. Vol. 2: The Criteria and Standards of Quality.* Ann Arbor, MI: Health Administration Press.

———. 1985. *Explorations in Quality Assessment and Monitoring. Vol. 3: The Methods and Findings of Quality Assessment and Monitoring: An Illustrated Analysis.* Ann Arbor, MI: Health Administration Press.

Dubay, L. 1989. *Changes in the Nursing Home Industry between 1981 and 1986.* Washington, D.C.: The Urban Institute.

Dubay, L., and J. Cohen. 1988. *The Effects of Cost Containment and Ownership on Nursing Home Costs, Case Mix, and Staffing.* Report #3585-02. Washington, D.C.: The Urban Institute.

Dunlop, B. 1979. *The Growth of Nursing Home Care.* Lexington, MA: D. C. Heath and Company.

Eastwood, E. 1990. "New Findings on Patients Needing Post-Hospital Care." *Blueprint* (Winter). New York, NY: United Hospital Fund.

Eisendorfer, C., D. Kessler, and A. Spector, eds. 1989. *Caring for the Elderly: Reshaping Health Policy.* Baltimore, MD: The Johns Hopkins University Press.

Ermann, D. 1990. "Rural Health Care: The Future of the Hospital." *Medical Care Review* 47(1):33–73.

Eubanks, P. 1989. "Geriatric Care Should Address Rehabilitation Needs." *Hospitals* 63(17):68.

Evashwick, C., and L. Weiss, eds. 1987. *Managing the Continuum of Care.* Rockville, MD: Aspen Publishers.

Finkler, S. 1987. "Cost Issues." In *Swing Beds: Assessing Flexible Health Care in Rural Communities*, edited by J. Wiener, pp. 42–63. Washington, D.C.: Brookings Institution.

Fitzgerald, J., P. Moore, and R. Dittus. 1988. "The Care of Elderly Patients with Hip Fracture: Changes since Implementation of the Prospective Payment System." *New England Journal of Medicine* 319(21):1392–97.

Foley, S., M. Zahn, R. Schlenker, and J. Johnson. 1984. *Case Mix Measures and Medicaid Nursing Home Payment Rate Determination in West Virginia, Ohio, and Maryland.* Denver, CO: Center for Health Services Research, University of Colorado Health Sciences Center.

Foley, W. 1989. "Integrating Case Mix Payment and Quality of Care." Presented at the ORSA/TIMS Joint National Meeting, 17 October, New York, NY.

Fries, B., D. Nerenz, S. Falcon, M. Ashcraft, and C. Lee. 1990. "A Classification System for Long-Staying Psychiatric Patients." *Medical Care* 28(4):311–23.

Fries, J. 1980. "Aging, Natural Death, and the Compression of Morbidity." *New England Journal of Medicine* 303(3):130–35.

Garrard, J., R. L. Kane, D. Radosevich, C. Skay, S. Arnold, L. Kepferle, S. McDermott, and J. Buchanan. 1990. "Impact of Geriatric Nurse Practitioners on Nursing-Home Residents' Functional Status, Satisfaction, and Discharge Outcomes." *Medical Care* 28(3):271–83.

Gillick, M. 1989. "Long-Term Care Options for the Frail Elderly." *Journal of the American Geriatrics Society* 37(12):1198–203.

Gist, J. 1989. *Options for the Public Financing of Long-Term Care.* AARP Report #8908. Washington, D.C.: American Association of Retired Persons.

Gornick, M., and M. Hall. 1988. "Trends in Medicare Use of Post-Hospital Care." *Health Care Financing Review* (Annual Supplement):27–38.

Grim, S. 1989. "Testimony Before the Ohio Public Health Council on Hospital-Based Subacute/Skilled Care and Emergency Rules §3701-12-233 and §3701-12-234," 15 March, Dayton, OH.

———. 1990. "Swing Beds: A Strategy in Rural Hospitals' Fight to Survive." *Healthcare Financial Management* 44(4):32–37.

Grimaldi, P., and T. Jazwiecki. 1987. *Case-Mix Payment Systems for Nursing Home Care.* Chicago, IL: Pluribus Press.

Grob, G. 1986. "The Social History of Medicine and Disease in America: Problems and Possibilities." In *The Medicine Show: Patients, Physicians and the Perplexities of the Health Revolution in Modern Society*, edited by P. Branca. New York, NY: Science History Publications/USA.

Guterman, S., P. Eggers, G. Riley, T. Greene, and S. Terrell. 1988. "The First 3 Years of Medicare Prospective Payment: An Overview." *Health Care Financing Review* 9(3):67–77.

Haber, C. 1983. *Beyond Sixty-Five: The Dilemma of Old Age in America's Past.* New York: Cambridge University Press.

Hammons, G., and L. Pawlson. 1989. "Physician Payment Reform: Implications for Geriatrics." *Journal of the American Geriatrics Society* 37(11):1084–91.

Harel, Z., and L. Noelker. 1978. *The Impact of Social Integration on the Well-Being and Survival of Institutionalized Aged.* Presented at the 31st Annual Meeting of the Gerontological Society of America, November, Dallas, TX.

Harrington, C., and L. Grant. 1988. *The Study of Regulation of Home Health Care Agencies in Two States: California and Missouri*. San Francisco, CA: Institute for Health and Aging, University of California at San Francisco.

Harrington, C., J. Swan, and L. Grant. 1988. "Nursing Home Bed Capacity in the States, 1978–86." *Health Care Financing Review* 9(4):81–97.

Hawes, C., and C. Phillips. 1986. "The Changing Structure of the Nursing Home Industry and the Impact of Ownership on Quality, Cost, and Access." In *For-Profit Enterprise in Health Care*, edited by B. Gray. Report of the Institute of Medicine (U.S.) Committee on Implications of For-Profit Enterprise in Health Care. Washington, D.C.: National Academy Press.

Health Care Financing Administration (HCFA). U.S. Department of Health and Human Services. 1982. *Medicare and Medicaid Program; Rural Hospitals: Provision of Long-Term Care Services (Swing-Bed Provision); Flexibility in Application of Standards* (42 CFR Parts 405, 435, 440, 442, and 447). *Federal Register* 47(139)31518–33.

———. 1985. *Medicare and Medicaid Programs; Utilization and Quality Control Peer Review Organization (PRO): Assumption of Medicare Review Functions and Coordination with Medicaid—Final Rules. Federal Register* 50(74):15312–74.

———. 1987. "National Health Expenditures, 1986–2000." *Health Care Financing Review* 8(4):1–36.

———. 1988a. *Medicare Program; Utilization and Quality Control Peer Review Program: Third Scope of Work for Peer Review Organizations. Federal Register* 53(176):35234–37.

———. 1988b. *Skilled Nursing Facility Care: Purpose and Intent of New Guidelines*. Baltimore, MD, 16 February.

———. 1989a. *Medicare and Medicaid; Requirements for Long Term Care Facilities* (42 CFR Parts 405, 442, 447, 483, 488, 489, and 498). *Federal Register* 54(21):5316–72.

———. 1989b. *Medicare Program; Swing-Bed Program Changes* (42 CFR Parts 413, 424, 482, and 483). *Federal Register* 54(172):37270–76.

———. 1989c. *1989 HCFA Statistics*. HCFA Pub. No. 03294. Baltimore, MD, September.

Hedrick, S., T. Koepsell, and T. Inui. 1989. "Meta-Analysis of Home-Care Effects on Mortality and Nursing-Home Placement." *Medical Care* 27(11):1015–26.

Helbing, C., and R. Keene. 1989. "Use and Cost of Short-Stay Hospital Inpatient Services under Medicare, 1986." *Health Care Financing Review* 10(3):109–22.

Hendriksen, C., E. Lund, and E. Stromgard. 1989. "Hospitalization of Elderly People: A 3-Year Controlled Trial." *Journal of the American Geriatrics Society* 37(2):117–22.

Holahan, J., L. Dubay, G. Kenney, P. Welch, C. Bishop, and A. Dor. 1989. "Should Medicare Compensate for Administratively Necessary Days?" *The Milbank Quarterly* 67(1):137–67.

Holahan, J., L. Dubay, G. Kenney, W. Welch, C. Bishop, A. Dor, and S. Laudicina. 1988. *Should Medicare Compensate Hospitals for Administratively Necessary Days?* Report #3710-01-05. Washington, D.C.: The Urban Institute.

Holahan, J., and M. Sulvetta. 1989. "Assessing Medicare Reimbursement Options for Skilled Nursing Facility Care." *Health Care Financing Review* 10(3):13–27.

Hughes, S. 1985. "Apples and Oranges? A review of Evaluations of Community-Based Long-Term Care." *Health Services Research* 20(4):261–87.

————. 1986. *Long-Term Care: Options in an Expanding Market.* Homewood, IL: Dow Jones–Irwin.

Hyman, H. 1977. *Health Regulation: Certificate of Need and 1122.* Germantown, MD: Aspen Systems Corporation.

Institute of Medicine (IOM). 1986. *Improving the Quality of Care in Nursing Homes.* Washington, D.C.: National Academy Press.

Kane, R. A., R. L. Kane, and L. Rubenstein. 1989. "Comprehensive Assessment of the Elderly Patient." Chapter 12 in *Health Care of the Elderly: An Information Synthesis,* edited by M. Petersen and D. While, pp. 475–519. Newbury Park, CA: Sage Publications.

Kane, R. A., R. L. Kane, S. Arnold, J. Garrard, S. McDermott, and L. Kepferle. 1988. "Geriatric Nurse Practitioners as Nursing Home Employees: Implementing the Role." *The Gerontologist* 28(4):469–77.

Kane, R. L. 1988a. "Beyond Caring: The Challenge to Geriatrics." *Journal of American Geriatrics Society* 36(5):467–75.

————. 1988b. *Natural History of Post-Acute Care for Medicare Beneficiaries.* Cooperative Agreement #17-C-98891/5-02 with the Health Care Financing Administration and the Office of the Assistant Secretary for Planning and Evaluation, DHHS. Minneapolis, MN: University of Minnesota, School of Public Health.

————. 1990. "Promoting the Art of the Possible in Long-Term Care." *American Journal of Public Health* 80(1):15–16.

Kane, R. L., J. Garrard, C. Skay, D. Radosevich, J. Buchanan, S. McDermott, S. Arnold, and L. Kepferle. 1989. "Effects of a Geriatric Nurse Practitioner on Process and Outcome of Nursing Home Care." *American Journal of Public Health* 79(9):1271–77.

Kane, R. L., J. Garrard, J. Buchanan, S. Arnold, R. A. Kane, and S. McDermott. 1989. "The Geriatric Nurse Practitioner as a Nursing Home Employee: Conceptual and Methodological Issues in Assessing Quality of Care and Cost Effectiveness." In *Nursing Homes and Nursing Care: Lessons from the Teaching Nursing Homes,* edited by M. Mezey, J. Lynaugh, and M. Cartier. New York, NY: Springer Publishing Company.

Kane, R. L., R. Bell, S. Riegler, A. Wilson, and E. Keeler. 1983. "Predicting the Outcomes of Nursing Home Patients." *The Gerontologist* 23(2):200–206.

Kane, R. L., and R. Matthias. 1984. "From Hospital to Nursing Home: The Long-Term Care Connection." *The Gerontologist* 24(6):604–9.

Kavesh, W., R. Mark, and B. Kearney. 1984. "Medical Care Teams Improve Nursing Home Care and Reduce Costs." Presented at the 37th Annual Scientific Meeting of the Gerontological Society of America, 16–20 November, San Antonio, TX.

Kayser-Jones, J., C. Wiener, and J. Barbaccia. 1989. "Factors Contributing to the Hospitalization of Nursing Home Residents." *The Gerontologist* 29(4):502–10.

Kemp, B., K. Brummel-Smith, and J. Ramsdell, eds. 1990. *Geriatric Rehabilitation.* Boston, MA: College-Hill Press.

Kemper, P., R. Applebaum, and M. Harrigan. 1987. "Community Care Demonstrations: What Have We Learned?" *Health Care Financing Review* 8(4):87–99.

Koff, S. 1988. *Health Systems Agencies: A Comprehensive Examination of Planning and Process.* New York, NY: Human Sciences Press.

Kovner, A., and H. Richardson. 1987. "Implementing Swing-Bed Services in Small Rural Hospitals." In *Medicare and Extended Care: Issues, Problems, and*

Prospects, edited by B. Vladeck and G. Alfano, pp. 91–107. A United Hospital Fund Book. Owings Mills, MD: National Health Publishing.

Kramer, A., P. Shaughnessy, and J. Stiles. 1989. *Transitional Care Provided in Skilled Nursing Facility Units in Acute Care Hospitals.* Denver, CO: Center for Health Services Research, University of Colorado Health Sciences Center.

Kurowski, B., and P. Shaughnessy. 1983. "The Measurement and Assurance of Quality." In *Long-Term Care: Perspectives from Research and Demonstrations,* edited by R. Vogel and H. Palmer. Washington, D.C.: U.S. Department of Health and Human Services, Health Care Financing Administration.

Landes, D., P. Shaughnessy, and E. Tynan; with E. Lutz, A. Woodson, C. Huggs, A. Jones, and B. Kurowski. 1979. *Swing-Bed Experiments to Provide Long-Term Care in Rural Hospitals in Iowa, South Dakota, and Texas: Final Report of the Quality Component of the Evaluation.* Denver, CO: Center for Health Services Research, University of Colorado Health Sciences Center.

Latta, V., and R. Keene. 1989. "Use and Cost of Skilled Nursing Facility Services under Medicare, 1987." *Health Care Financing Review* 11(1):105–16.

Lave, J., and L. Lave. 1974. *The Hospital Construction Act: An Evaluation of the Hill-Burton Program, 1948–1973.* Washington, D.C.: American Enterprise Institute for Public Policy Research.

Lefton, E., S. Bonstelle, and J. Frengley. 1983. "Success with an Inpatient Geriatric Unit: A Controlled Study of Outcome and Follow-Up." *Journal of the American Geriatrics Society* 31(3):149–55.

Letsch, S., K. Levit, and D. Waldo. 1988. "National Health Expenditures, 1987." *Health Care Financing Review* 10(2):109–22.

Lewin/ICF. 1988. *Subacute Care in Hospitals: Synthesis of Findings from the 1987 Survey of Hospitals and Case Studies in Five States.* Prepared for the Prospective Payment Assessment Commission. Technical Report No. E-88-01, September.

Lewis, M., B. Leake, V. Clark, and M. Leal-Sotelo. 1990. "Changes in Case Mix and Outcomes of Readmissions to Nursing Homes between 1980 and 1984." *Health Services Research* 24(6):713–28.

Lipson, D., and C. Thomas. 1986. *State Regulation of Subacute Care: A 50 State Survey.* Washington, D.C.: Intergovernmental Health Policy Project, The George Washington University.

Liu, K., and K. Manton. 1988. *Effects of Medicare's Hospital Prospective Payment System (PPS) on Disabled Medicare Beneficiaries.* Final Report. Washington, D.C.: The Urban Institute.

Liu, K., P. Doty, and K. Manton. 1990. "Medicaid Spenddown in Nursing Homes." *The Gerontologist* 30(1):7–15.

Lohr, K., and S. Schroeder. 1990. "Special Report: A Strategy for Quality Assurance in Medicare." *New England Journal of Medicine* 322(10)707–12.

Lyles, Y. 1986. "Impact of Medicare Diagnosis-Related Groups (DRGs) on Nursing Homes in the Portland, Oregon Metropolitan Area." *Journal of the American Geriatrics Society* 34(8):573–78.

Mariano, L. 1989. "Growth of the Medicare Population." *Health Care Financing Review* 10(3):123–24.

Master, R., M. Feltin, J. Jainshill, R. Mark, W. Kavesh, M. Rabkin, B. Turner, S. Bachrach, and S. Lennox. 1980. "A Continuum of Care for the Inner City: Assessment of Its Benefits for Boston's Elderly and High Risk Population." *New England Journal of Medicine* 302(26):1434–40.

McCusker, J., D. Mundt, A. Stoddard, E. Cole, and S. Whitbourne. 1989. "Outcomes of a Geriatric Rehabilitation Program in a Long-Term Care Facility." *Journal of Aging and Health* 1(4):485–506.

Mendelson, M. 1974. *Tender Loving Greed: How the Incredibly Lucrative Nursing Home "Industry" is Exploiting America's Old People and Defrauding Us All.* New York, NY: Alfred A. Knopf.

Merrill, J., and S. Somers. 1989. "Long-Term Care: The Great Debate on the Wrong Issue." *Inquiry* 267(3):317–20.

Mickel, C. 1989. "Excess Capacity Becomes Center of Policy Debate." *Hospitals* 63(17):38–43.

Migdail, K., ed. 1989. "New Benefits Cause Medicare SNF Costs to Skyrocket." *Long Term Care Management* 18(17):1.

Mitchell, J. 1978. "Patient Outcomes in Alternative Long-Term Settings." *Medical Care* 16(6):439–52.

Mitchell, S. 1989. *Subacute Care in Minnesota Hospitals, 1987.* St. Paul, MN: Minnesota Department of Health.

Moon, M. 1985. "Evaluability Assessment of the Medicare Prospective Payment System on Long-Term Care." In *Preliminary Analyses on Medicare PPS and Long-Term Care,* edited by M. Sulvetta. Washington, D.C.: The Urban Institute.

———. 1989. "Taking the Plunge: The Arguments for a Comprehensive Long-Term Care System." *Journal of the American Geriatrics Society* 37(12):1165–70.

Morishita, L., A. Siu, R. Wang, C. Oken, M. Cadogan, and L. Schwartzman. 1989. "Comprehensive Geriatric Care in a Day Hospital: A Demonstration of the British Model in the U.S." *The Gerontologist* 29(3):336–40.

Moroney, R., and N. Kurtz. 1975. "The Evolution of Long-Term Care Institutions." In *Long-Term Care: A Handbook for Researchers, Planners, and Providers,* edited by S. Sherwood. New York, NY: Spectrum Publications.

Morrisey, M., F. Sloan, and J. Valvona. 1988. "Shifting Medicare Patients Out of the Hospital." *Health Affairs* 7(5):52–64.

Moscovice, I. 1989. "Rural Hospitals: A Literature Synthesis and Health Services Research Agenda." *Health Services Research* 23(6):891–903.

Moses, S. 1990. "The Fallacy of Impoverishment." *The Gerontologist* 30(1):21–25.

Moss, F., and V. Halamandaris. 1977. *Too Old, Too Sick, Too Bad: Nursing Homes in America.* Germantown, MD: Aspen Systems Corporation.

National Center for Health Studies (NCHS). 1988. *Health, United States, 1987.* DHHS Pub. No. (PHS) 88-1232. Public Health Service. Washington, D.C.: U.S. Government Printing Office.

Neu, C., and S. Harrison. 1988. *Posthospital Care Before and After the Medicare Prospective Payment System.* Santa Monica, CA: The RAND Corporation.

New York State Department of Health and Rensselaer Polytechnic Institute. 1984. *New York State Long-Term Care Case Mix Reimbursement Project, Executive Summary: Derivation of RUG-II.* New York, NY, December.

North Dakota State Health Council. 1989. *An Evaluation of Swing Beds in North Dakota.* Bismarck, ND: State Health Council, North Dakota Department of Health and Consolidated Laboratories, Division of Health Resource Analysis.

Oregon Association of Hospitals. 1986. *Position Paper: Sub-Acute Care.* Portland, OR: Oregon Association of Hospitals.

Pauly, M., and P. Wilson. 1986. "Hospital Outpatient Forecasts and the Cost of Empty Beds." *Health Services Research* 21(3):403–28.

Pennell, F. 1982. "Reimbursement: 'Carve-out' Method Benefits Swing-Bed Hospitals." *Hospitals* 56(22):79–84.

Polich, C., L. Secord, and M. Parker. 1986. *Transitional Care: A Report on Minnesota's Experience.* Minneapolis, MN: Minnesota Association of Homes for the Aging, Minnesota Hospital Association, and InterStudy.

Prospective Payment Assessment Commission (ProPAC). 1986. "Appendix C: Cross-Cutting Issues—Peer Review Organizations: Mission and Function." In *Technical Appendices to the Report and Recommendations to the Secretary,* U.S. Department of Health and Human Services, pp. 157–62. Washington, D.C.: U.S. Government Printing Office.

————. 1988. *Medicare Prospective Payment System and the American Health Care System Report to Congress.* Chicago, IL: Commerce Business Clearing House.

Read, W., and J. O'Brien. 1989. "The Involved Hospital." In *Caring for the Elderly: Reshaping Health Policy,* edited by C. Eisdorfer, D. Kessler, and A. Spector. Baltimore, MD: The Johns Hopkins University Press.

Reed, S., and J. Gessner. 1979. "Rehabilitation in the Extended Care Facility." *Journal of the American Geriatrics Society* 27(7):325–29.

Richardson, H., and A. Kovner. 1985. "Update on the National Swing-Bed Demonstration." *Kentucky Hospitals* 2(11):20–22.

————. 1986. "Implementing Swing-Bed Services in Small Rural Hospitals." *Journal of Rural Health* 2(1):46–60.

————. 1987. "Swing-Beds: Current Experience and Future Directions." *Health Affairs* 6(3):61–74.

Rivlin, A., and J. Wiener; with R. Hanley, and D. Spence. 1988. *Caring for the Disabled Elderly: Who Will Pay?* Washington, D.C.: Brookings Institution.

Rosenberg, C. 1977. "And Heal the Sick: Hospitals and Patients in 19th Century America." In *The Medicine Show,* edited by P. Branca. New York, NY: Science History Publications.

Rowe, J. 1985. "Health Care of the Elderly." *New England Journal of Medicine* 312(13):827–35.

Rubenstein, L., I. Abrass, and R. L. Kane. 1981. "Improved Care for Patients on a New Geriatric Evaluation Unit." *Journal of the American Geriatrics Society* 29(11):531–36.

Rubenstein, L., K. Josephson, G. Wieland, P. English, J. Sagre, and R. L. Kane. 1984. "Effectiveness of a Geriatric Evaluation Unit." *New England Journal of Medicine* 311(26):1664–70.

Rubenstein, L., L. Rhee, and R. L. Kane. 1982. "The Role of Geriatric Assessment Units in Caring for the Elderly: An Analytic Review." *Journal of Gerontology* 37(5):513–21.

Ruther, M., and C. Helbing. 1988. "Use and Cost of Home Health Agency Services under Medicare." *Health Care Financing Review* 10(1):105–8.

Safran, D., and E. Eastwood. 1989. *Transitional Care: The Problem of Alternate Level of Care in New York City.* New York, NY: United Hospital Fund.

Sager, M., E. Leventhal, and D. Easterling. 1987. "The Impact of Medicare's Prospective Payment System on Wisconsin Nursing Homes." *Journal of the American Medical Association* 257(13):1762–66.

Sankar, A., R. Newcomer, and J. Wood. 1986. "Prospective Payment: Systemic Effects on the Provision of Community Care for the Elderly." *Home Health Care Services Quarterly* 7(2):93–117.

Scanlon, W. 1988. "A Perspective on Long-Term Care for the Elderly." *Health Care Financing Review* (Annual Supplement):7–15.

Schlenker, R. 1988. *An Analysis of Long-Term Care Payment Systems, Executive*

Summary. Denver, CO: Center for Health Services Research, University of Colorado Health Sciences Center.

Schlenker, R.; with J. Stiles, T. Carlough, and P. DeVore. 1988. *A Multi-State Analysis of Medicaid Nursing Home Payment Systems.* Denver, CO: Center for Health Services Research, University of Colorado Health Sciences Center.

Schlenker, R., and P. Shaughnessy. 1989. "Swing-Bed Hospital Cost and Reimbursement." *Inquiry* 26(4):508–21.

Schuman, J., E. Beattie, D. Steed, J. Gibson, G. Merry, W. Campbell, and A. Kraus. 1978. "The Impact of a New Geriatric Program in a Hospital for the Chronically Ill." *Canadian Medical Association Journal* 118(6):639–45.

Seifer, S. 1987. "The Impact of PPS on Home Health Care: A Survey of Thirty-Five Home Health Agencies." *Caring* 6(4):10–12.

Seksenski, E. 1987. "Discharges from Nursing Homes: Preliminary Data from the 1985 National Nursing Home Survey." In *Advance Data from Vital and Health Statistics.* National Center for Health Statistics. No. 142. DHHS Pub. No. (PHS)87-1250. Hyattsville, MD: U.S. Public Health Service.

Shapiro, E., and R. Tate. 1989. "Is Health Care Use Changing? A Comparison between Physician, Hospital, Nursing-Home, and Home-Care Use of Two Elderly Cohorts." *Medical Care* 27(11):1002–14.

Shaughnessy, P. 1978. "The Road to Survival: Saving the Rural Hospital—The Need Is There, Diversification Is the Means." *Hospital Forum* 21(5):16–18, 22.

———. 1984. "Overview of Swing-Bed Care." In *A Swing-Bed Planning Guide for Rural Hospitals,* edited by J. Supplitt. Chicago, IL: American Hospital Publishing.

———. 1987. "Access and Case-Mix Patterns." In *Brookings Dialogues in Public Policy: Swing Beds, Assessing Flexible Health Care in Rural Communities,* edited by J. Wiener. Washington, D.C.: Brookings Institution.

———. 1989. "Quality of Nursing Home Care." *Generations* 13(1):17–20.

Shaughnessy, P., A. Jones, C. Huggs, D. Landes, E. Tynan, K. Paulson, B. Kurowski, and J. Lubitz. 1978a. *A Swing-Bed Experiment to Provide Long-Term Care in Rural Hospitals in Utah, Volume I.* Denver, CO: Center for Health Services Research, Office of the Chancellor for Health Affairs, University of Colorado Medical Center.

———. 1978b. *A Swing-Bed Experiment to Provide Long-Term Care in Rural Hospitals in Utah, Volume II.* Denver, CO: Center for Health Services Research, Office of the Chancellor for Health Affairs, University of Colorado Medical Center.

Shaughnessy, P., and A. Kramer. 1990. "The Increased Needs of Patients in Nursing Homes and Patients Receiving Home Health Care." *New England Journal of Medicine* 322(1):21–27.

Shaughnessy, P., A. Kramer, and D. Hittle. 1990. *The Teaching Nursing Home Experiment: It's Effects and Implications.* Denver, CO: Center for Health Services Research, University of Colorado Health Sciences Center.

Shaughnessy, P., A. Kramer, and M. Pettigrew; with J. Stiles, D. Vahling, M. Brown, A. McFarlane, II, S. Graff, and P. DeVore. 1987. *Findings on Case Mix and Quality of Care in Nursing Homes and Home Health Agencies.* Denver, CO: Center for Health Services Research, University of Colorado Health Sciences Center.

Shaughnessy, P., A. Kramer, R. Schlenker, and M. Polesovsky. 1985. "Nursing Home Case-Mix Differences between Medicare and Non-Medicare and between Hospital-Based and Freestanding Patients." *Inquiry* 22(2):162–77.

Shaughnessy, P., C. Huggs, D. Landes, and E. Tynan. 1979. *Swing-Bed Experiments to Provide Long-Term Care in Rural Hospitals in Iowa, South Dakota, and Texas: Second Year Report*. Denver, CO: Center for Health Services Research, University of Colorado Health Sciences Center.

Shaughnessy, P., E. Tynan, D. Landes, C. Huggs, D. Holub, and L. Breed. 1980a. *An Evaluation of Swing-Bed Experiments to Provide Long-Term Care in Rural Hospitals, Volume I: Final Summary Report*. Denver, CO: Center for Health Services Research, University of Colorado Health Sciences Center.

———. 1980b. *An Evaluation of Swing-Bed Experiments to Provide Long-Term Care in Rural Hospitals, Volume II: Final Technical Report*. Denver, CO: Center for Health Services Research, University of Colorado Health Sciences Center.

Shaughnessy, P., L. Breed, and D. Landes. 1982. "Assessing the Quality of Care Provided in Rural Swing-Bed Hospitals." *Quality Review Bulletin* 8(5):12–20.

Shaughnessy, P., and R. Schlenker. 1986. "Hospital Swing-Bed Care in the United States." *Health Services Research* 21(4):477–98.

Shaughnessy, P., and R. Schlenker; with C. Braunstein, D. Hittle, S. Harden, M. Spencer, D. Vahling, W. Grant, D. Beck, and C. Pace. 1985. *Hospital Swing Beds in the United States: Initial Findings*. Denver, CO: Center for Health Services Research, University of Colorado Health Sciences Center.

Shaughnessy, P., and R. Schlenker; with D. Hittle, J. Stiles, T. Carlough, and W. Grant. 1988. *Rural Acute and Postacute Care under Medicare's Prospective Payment System*. Denver, CO: Center for Health Services Research, University of Colorado Health Sciences Center.

Shaughnessy, P., R. Schlenker, and A. Kramer. 1990. "Quality of Long-Term Care in Nursing Homes and Swing-Bed Hospitals." *Health Services Research* 25, no. 1 (Part 1):65–96.

Shaughnessy, P., R. Schlenker, and D. Hittle; with S. Harden, M. Spencer, D. Beck, D. Vahling, W. Grant, L. Mason, J. McGloin, J. Amirani, A. McFarlane, II, S. Graff, P. DeVore, and W. Van Epps. 1989a. *Hospital Swing Beds: A Study of Long-Term Care Provided in Acute Care Beds in Rural America, 1982–1986, Volume I: Summary Report*. Denver, CO: Center for Health Services Research, University of Colorado Health Sciences Center.

———. 1989b. *Hospital Swing Beds: A Study of Long-Term Care Provided in Acute Care Beds in Rural America, 1982–1986, Volume II: Technical Report*. Denver, CO: Center for Health Services Research, University of Colorado Health Sciences Center.

Shaughnessy, P., R. Schlenker, and M. Polesovsky. 1986. "Medicaid and Non-Medicaid Case Mix Differences in Colorado Nursing Homes." *Medical Care* 24(6):482–95.

Shortell, S., and W. McNerney. 1990. "The Future of the American Health Care System." *New England Journal of Medicine* 322(7):463–66.

Silverman, H. 1989. "Reports to Congress: Review of Swing-Bed Care by Peer Review Organizations." *Health Care Financing Review* 11(2):137.

———. 1990. "Medicare Reimbursement for Swing-Bed Hospitals." *Health Care Financing Review* 11(3):99–106.

Sloan, F., M. Morrisey, and J. Valvona. 1988a. "Effects of the Medicare Prospective Payment System on Hospital Cost Containment: An Early Appraisal." *The Milbank Quarterly* 66(2):191–220.

———. 1988b. "Medicare Prospective Payment and the Use of Medical Technologies in Hospitals." *Medical Care* 26(9):837–50.

Smeeding, T. 1990. "Editorial: Toward a Knowledge Base for Long-Term Care Finance." *The Gerontologist* 30(1):5–6.

Solomon, D. 1988. "Geriatric Assessment: Methods for Clinical Decision Making." *Journal of the American Medical Association* 295(16):2450–52.

Spence, D., and J. Wiener. 1990. "Nursing Home Length of Stay Patterns: Results from the 1985 National Nursing Home Survey." *The Gerontologist* 30(1):16–20.

Supplitt, J. 1982. "Swing Beds: New Diversification Opportunity for Small and Rural Hospitals." *Hospitals* 56(22):67–72.

———. 1984. *A Swing-Bed Planning Guide for Rural Hospitals*. Chicago, IL: American Hospital Publishing.

Timmreck, T. 1989. "Subacute Care in Long-Term Care Facilities." *The Journal of Long-Term Care Administration* (Summer):14–17.

Tobin, S., and R. Kulys. 1980. "The Family and Services." In *Annual Review of Gerontology and Geriatrics*, edited by C. Eisendorfer. New York, NY: Springer Publishing Company.

Townsend, C. 1971. *Old Age: The Last Segregation.* New York, NY: Grossman Publishers.

Trisel, B. 1988. *An Analysis of Subaute Care in Ohio*. Columbus, OH: Ohio Department of Health.

U.S. Congress. House. Select Committee on Aging. 1985. *America's Elderly at Risk*. Washington, D.C.: U.S. Government Printing Office.

U.S. Congress. House. 1989. "Quicker and Sicker: Substandard Treatment of Medicare Patients (HR 101-387)." Seventh Report by the Committee on Government Operations Together with Additional Views. Washington, D.C.: U.S. Government Printing Office.

U.S. Congress. Office of Technology Assessment (OTA). 1990. *Health Care in Rural America*. OTA-H-434. Washington, D.C.: U.S. Government Printing Office, September.

U.S. Congress. Senate. Special Committee on Aging. 1974. *Nursing Home Care in the United States: Failure in Public Policy.* Subcommittee on Long-Term Care. Washington, D.C.: U.S. Government Printing Office.

———. 1984. *Senate Hearing 98-1091 on Discrimination against the Poor and Disabled in Nursing Homes*. 98th Cong., 2d. Sess. Washington, D.C.: U.S. Government Printing Office.

———. 1986a. *Crisis in Home Health Care: Greater Need, Less Care*. Serial No. 99-24. Washington, D.C.: U.S. Government Printing Office.

———. 1986b. *Nursing Home Care: The Unfinished Agenda*. Washington, D.C.: U.S. Government Printing Office.

U.S. Department of Health, Education, and Welfare (DHEW). 1977. *Health Insurance Statistics*, HI-75. Washington, D.C.: U.S. Government Printing Office.

———. 1978. *New Directions for Skilled Nursing and Intermediate Care Facilities: Summaries of Public Hearings, June–August 1978*. Rockville, MD: Health Care Financing Administration.

U.S. General Accounting Office (GAO). 1983. *Medicaid and Nursing Home Care: Cost Increases and the Need for Services are Creating Problems for the States and the Elderly.* Report to the Chairman of the Subcommittee on Health and the Environment, Committee on Energy and Commerce, House of Representatives. Washington, D.C.: U.S. Government Printing Office.

———. 1987. *Medicare and Medicaid: Stronger Enforcement of Nursing Home Require-*

ments Needed. Report to the Ranking Minority Member, Special Committee on Aging, U.S. Senate Publication No. GAO/HRD-87-113. Washington, D.C.: U.S. Government Printing Office.

————. 1988. *Medicare: Improving Quality of Care Assessment and Assurance*. Report to the Chairman, Subcommittee on Health, Committee on Ways and Means, House of Representatives. GAO/PEMD-88-10. Washington, D.C.: U.S. Government Printing Office.

Vladeck, B. 1980. *Unloving Care: The Nursing Home Tragedy*. New York, NY: Basic Books.

————. 1987a. "The Meaning of the Swing-Bed Experience." In *Swing Beds: Assessing Flexible Health Care in Rural Communities*, edited by J. Wiener. Washington, D.C.: Brookings Institution.

————. 1987b. "The Continuum of Care: Principles and Metaphors." In *Managing the Continuum of Care*, edited by C. Evashwick and L. Weiss. Rockville, MD: Aspen Publishers.

————. 1988. "Hospital Prospective Payment and the Quality of Care." *New England Journal of Medicine* 319(21):1411–13.

Vladeck, B., and G. Alfano. 1987. *Medicare and Extended Care: Issues, Problems, and Prospects*. A United Hospital Fund Book. Owings Mills, MD: National Health Publishing.

Vogel, D. 1980. *The Invention of the Modern Hospital: Boston, 1870–1930*. Chicago, IL: University of Chicago Press.

Waldo, D., K. Levit, and H. Lazenby. 1986. "National Health Expenditures, 1985." *Health Care Financing Review* 8(1):1–21.

Weiner, S., J. Maxwell, H. Sapolsky, D. Dunn, and W. Hsaio. 1987. "Economic Incentives and Organizational Realities: Managing Hospitals under DRGs." *The Milbank Quarterly* 65(4):463–87.

Weissert, W. 1985. "Estimating the Long-Term Care Population: Prevalence Rates and Selected Characteristics." *Health Care Financing Review* 6(4):83–91.

Weissert, W., C. Cready, and J. Pawelak. 1988. "Past and Future of Home- and Community-Based Long-Term Care." *The Milbank Quarterly* 66(2):309–88.

Wiener, J., ed. 1987. *Swing Beds: Assessing Flexible Health Care in Rural Communities*. Washington, D.C.: Brookings Institution.

Williams, M., T. Williams, J. Zimmer, W. Hall, and C. Podgorski. 1987. "How Does the Team Approach to Outpatient Geriatric Evaluation Compare with Traditional Care: A Report of a Randomized Controlled Trial." *Journal of the American Geriatrics Society* 35(12):1071–78.

Williamson, J. 1989. "The Need for a Geriatrics Specialty: Lessons from the United Kingdom." In *Caring for the Elderly: Reshaping Health Policy*, edited by C. Eisdorfer, D. Kessler, and A. Spector. Baltimore, MD: The Johns Hopkins University Press.

Zimmer, J., G. Eggert, A. Treat, and B. Brodows. 1988. "Nursing Homes as Acute Care Providers: A Pilot Study of Incentives to Reduce Hospitalizations." *Journal of the American Geriatrics Society* 36(2):124–29.

Index

About the Author

Peter W. Shaughnessy, Ph.D., is director of the Center for Health Services Research at the University of Colorado Health Sciences Center. His doctorate is in mathematics with an emphasis in probability theory and mathematical statistics. He has taught courses and seminars in health policy and health policy research, program evaluation and research methods, case-mix and quality measurement, and statistical inference and quantitative decision making. Professor Shaughnessy's primary faculty appointment is in the Department of Medicine at the University of Colorado School of Medicine, with joint appointments in the School of Nursing and the Health Administration Program in the School of Business. Prior to establishing the Center for Health Services Research at the University of Colorado 15 years ago, he conducted health care research at the National Institutes of Health, National Center for Health Statistics, and other private organizations. His interest in integrating research, programmatic, clinical, and financing issues and approaches in health care has resulted in lectures and presentations to a variety of practitioner, policy-oriented, and academic audiences.

Dr. Shaughnessy's publications are largely in the areas of health policy, long-term care, hospital care, research methods, and applications involving the measurement of cost, case mix, and quality of care in health services research. He has published widely in journals such as the *Journal of the American Statistical Association, Health Services Research, New England Journal of Medicine, Health Care Financing Review, Inquiry,* and *Medical Care.* His experience includes memberships on the editorial board of *Health Services Research,* various grant review panels, advisory committees of several national health policy studies, and the board of directors of the Association of Health Services Research. He also served on the Committee for Nursing Home Regulation at the National Academy of Sciences' Institute of Medicine. During the past 20 years, he has been principal investigator on nine multi-year national studies to assess the cost and quality of long-term care as provided by nursing homes, home health agencies, and hospitals.